Healer: The Jerry Wills Story

Rod Haberer

Cover Photo by Kathy Wills

ISBN-13: 978-1494391812
ISBN-10: 1494391813

DEDICATION

To Jerry and Kathy Wills without whom this book would never have been possible. And to all the people Jerry has helped for sharing their stories. And for my wife Ellen, for her patience and love.

CONTENTS

Introduction

Pain. Some believe it's just a state of mind. And in fact, it is. Pain is the way our body communicates a problem. "Hey," it says, "something's wrong down here." Or, "Ouch, I'm hurt!" after an unfortunate accident.

Pain is powerful. Many people fear pain more than they fear death.

Anytime someone is injured or doesn't feel well, he or she usually turns to the ways of western medicine. It begins with a call to the doctor's office, or maybe a trip to the emergency room. If you have a broken leg or a fever of more than 103 degrees, you might get to see a doctor right away. Otherwise, it will be hours – maybe a regular appointment with your doctor a week or two away. We all know the drill.

Once you get to see your doctor, you may leave with an X-ray slip for further diagnosis. If you are lucky, you just get a prescription for pain medication and maybe an antibiotic for infection.

Over the years, I've seen people in pain. Some were strangers. Others were people I love. A few of them decided to try something different to ease the suffering. They went to an energy or faith healer…like Jerry Wills. Some people call Jerry an "Energy Healer" or "Faith Healer." Jerry prefers the term "Intuitive Healer." Still others like myself choose the simpler "Healer." By whatever name you choose, Jerry Wills apparently has the ability to "see" what ails a person and to manipulate human tissue at a cellular level to repair the damage. But it's really much more than that.

I've seen Jerry work on people. Most showed immediate improvement. For others, it takes longer. Jerry says he can help, if it is his and the client's destiny to heal. Usually it is.

Healing the way Jerry does is about turning desperation into hope—an act of goodness that transcends the physical world as we know it. Even after spending months with Jerry in preparation for writing this book, I still don't know how he does it. I only know that I look at medical problems differently now.

But let's get things straight here – I am a non-believer, a skeptic of the highest order. I still am. I've been a broadcast news journalist for twenty-nine years. News people are genetically skeptical of all things – we don't believe anything we are told, at first. I went into this project with a very skeptical attitude, but an open mind. I have a show-me feeling about things; if I can see it with my own eyes, if I can see the work repeated over and over, and if I can be convinced there is a rational explanation no matter how far fetched, then it is something worth learning more about.

In any case, don't take my word for it. Read the book. I believe I did my best to bring you, the reader, a very straight forward story based on interviews with Jerry, other healers, internationally known researchers, and Jerry's clients. This is not an effort to convince you that energy healing is real. On the other hand, neither is this book an investigative work about energy healing. It's based only on first hand accounts and interviews I conducted over many months.

Neither did I write about "the truth" when it comes to energy healing. The reason is simple. Truth depends on your point of view – something I've learned after receiving a few hundred thousand viewer phone calls over the years. The truth is what you make of it – I'm not going to do it for you.

I'm also not out to expose fraud. It's too big a task. There have been some fascinating examples of how some unscrupulous people have, and still are, defrauding people of money by posing as faith healers. You've probably already heard about a few. But keep one thing in mind. Fraud is everywhere, in every profession. There are lawyers who defraud their clients of millions of dollars every year. There are doctors who defraud Medicare and other insurance providers by over-billing or over-charging patients' insurance companies, or practice medicine without a license. There are construction workers who take money but never finish the job. But at the same time there are honest doctors who do their best to help people, good lawyers who protect the rights of their clients and construction workers who finish the job on time and under budget.

Simply put, fraud is as old as time. By the same token, there are honest people sincerely trying to provide a service that helps people at a fair price. Just because there is fraud in faith healing, does that necessarily mean all faith healers are frauds? You'll have to make up your own mind about healers like Jerry Wills. Just consider the fact that maybe, just maybe, there is something more than fraud at work here.

After you read this book, ask your own questions. It's how we learn. It is also how we open our minds to possibilities we never dreamed of.

As for Jerry, he is a mostly private man – he seeks neither fame nor fortune. And he is the first to admit that his talents cannot help everyone.

Although Jerry recently established a rate for his service, no one is turned away. Some more financially fortunate people he has helped provide an income that help Jerry with his necessities, and help him help others who can't pay. It's a development that also allows Jerry to work as a healer full time now, instead of supplementing his income, which primarily came from his work as an electronics technician. That's what Jerry was doing when I first met him – repairing TV's and VCR's for a living, while helping people for free.

For a healer to charge anything at all is heresy to many people. A "Laying on of Hands" as some people call it should never come with financial strings attached. But ask yourself this question. If Jerry worked full time as a healer, how would he eat? How would he live if he didn't charge a fee? We are no longer living in Biblical times. This is the 21st century. Unless you plan on living in a cardboard box under a freeway overpass, you have to have money. So now Jerry has a base fee for his services.

When most people think of healers, the mega-televangelists come to mind. Not someone like Jerry. Many mega-ministries have 100,000 people attend their traveling shows, and everyone's throwing money into the pot. Their organizations walk away with a half million dollars or more. But to Jerry, it's not about the money. He said, "I wish I didn't have to worry about the money. If I had money in the bank coming from some other source, and someone calls saying they need help, a set fee for my services would not be part of this equation. I would simply request they give me something, whatever they could afford or think is right. But that's not my reality."

At the time this book is being published, Jerry and his wife Kathy rent an apartment in Jerome, Arizona, north of Phoenix. But in between short stays they travel from city to city, state to state and sometimes country to country trying to help people who can at least pay their expenses to wherever Jerry's next client lives.

After meeting Jerry, one thing was perfectly clear. Jerry's need for income is secondary to his desire to help people – another reason I chose him for this book. Unlike some healers, Jerry's work is clearly not tainted by greed. He leaves the theatrics and riches to others. Jerry truly wants to help people. He thinks goodness and kindness are their own rewards – providing a lifetime of happy memories.

Try it yourself. Think back to a time when you were kind to someone. Makes you feel good, doesn't it? It's something that happens to Jerry on a daily basis – several times a day, in fact. Wouldn't that be worth something to you? It is to Jerry.

Call it what you will. A Miracle is one way. Energy healing is another. Not even Jerry can share everything about his life and his abilities to heal.

After spending days and days with Jerry and even more time watching him work on people, I feel I have a pretty good idea of what is going on. And I'll do my best to explain it to you. In this introduction, I'd like to give you a quick look at what Jerry does, how he explains it, and what the normal result is.

When Jerry meets someone for the first time, someone who requires his services, Jerry has certain hurdles he must cross.

Most of the time, his clients have already seen a regular doctor, who may have prescribed certain medicines or treatments for whatever ails his or her patient.

Because Jerry is not a doctor, he doesn't even ask what doctors have diagnosed, or what they call the problem his client has. Since he's not a doctor, he can't call or diagnose an illness by the words used by the medical profession. He might end up in legal hot water that way.

"The medical community has come up with a certain list of names," Jerry said in one of our many discussions. "Cancer, diabetes, arthritis, you know, and every so often a whole new list of words are added to this. These words are protected words. America is supposed to be the icon in the entire world for free speech, but it turns out that these words are protected and not free! So I have to be aware of the words that I'm using."

Jerry cites a past example: "A woman came to see me recently. Her back was hurting terribly. Her physician told her she has arthritis in her back, in her spine. So how do I address that? I simply address that she has pain in her back. I'm speaking to her with an awareness of what's going on and to her cause of this pain consciously. She and I both know the medical community commonly calls this condition arthritis. What do I call it? An inflamed area where the energy isn't properly focused or flowing? Arthritis is just a term, one for what I see happening. It is just a word defining a symptom, not an answer to why the condition exists. People come in and say I've got a tumor on my lung, and the doctors say it's cancer. Okay, what do I call that? Of course, I'm stepping over the line if I call it what they call it. For me, these 'words' are only medical descriptions. I respect the domain of the trained professionals who use them. For myself, I would much rather look for the cause and leave the terms to someone else."

When it comes to meeting a client for the first time, Jerry wants to know what they feel is wrong, not what their doctors think. "It's easy enough to just walk around and spout off what you've been told – oh, I've got this wrong and that wrong – these are the definitions that you're trying to convey to me that you've been told are wrong with you. But once I touch you and look inside to find answers that are meaningful to my understanding, I'm going to ask you a few questions. 'What do you think is wrong? How do you feel about it? What are you feeling? I want to know what it is inside of you that's saying there's something wrong and I need help. Is it because someone told you there is, or do you feel like there is?' Answering these questions honestly is when you start breaking into what's going on with a person. Some things are pretty common; a bone spur is a bone spur, a pain in the back, is a pain in the back. Whether you give it a clinical name, or it's a pain in the back, your personal experience remains the same!"

To Jerry, it's all about getting to the root cause of the person's discomfort, and then finding a way, his way, to heal it.

When people want to see Jerry it's usually because they have exhausted conventional medicine, and are unhappy with the outcome of treatment they have received. They are not all at the end of their rope, but often they are.

Jerry always greets someone very warmly. His six-foot-nine inch frame can be alarming to some, but his gentle manner and soft pleasant voice are immediately disarming and somehow trusting.

After a short greeting and discussion of their problem, Jerry always gets his client's permission to proceed. After granting permission, Jerry then asks them to relax, and to take several deep breaths. This usually calms the person Jerry is working on so he can move on.

Jerry then enters what I can only describe as a trance like state. He begins by closing his eyes, and bringing his hands together or closing them near his face. "I bring my hands up with my eyes closed," Jerry told me. "I can still see my hands even though my eyes are closed. As I breathe, and I breathe slowly, I bring my hands before my closed eyes. Within a short time, maybe a few seconds, I can see they're starting to glow. They look dark at first. Then they start getting this bluish white glow around them. Once I see this I'm ready to begin."

Jerry says he then enters a state that allows him to "see" his client in a way most people never can. He can see a field of energy that flows around and through them. He can also "see" their hopes, fears and secrets, but usually filters that out. His only concern is for the reason they have come to see him.

Jerry is ready to examine his client now. First, he holds his or her hands.

Most of the time, Jerry sees the problem right away. "Whether it's hair follicles, or veins and arteries, nerves, bones, connective tissue or whatever it is, it just lights up for me," he said. "As I'm sitting there holding their hands, everything just sort of comes up to a glow."

At this point, Jerry says everything begins to change. "I go very deep into a realm where I'm not really aware of the room I'm in, people who might be there or things nearby. Instead, the energy flowing through me is drawing me into the body of the person I am sitting with. A way to describe this is to say I've just entered into a vivid movie where I can look around and interact with my surroundings. My client has told me what they think is wrong, I've usually been told what the doctors think is wrong, now my energy is moving all through this person's body, touching everything."

"Within moments I have seen where something seems out of place. Healthy areas glow very brightly. Distressed areas do not." Jerry continued. "It's at that point I can see what's really wrong with them versus what they think or have been told is wrong. Sometimes it is the same thing. Often there are other issues causing the distress and contributing to what the condition seems to be. Sometimes my client is aware of these other issues; sometimes they are not. Once I've finished this process, which only takes just a few minutes, I let go of their hands. The return rush of energy sometimes causes me take a deep breath when I disconnect. Once it comes rushing back in to me, that's when I usually go…whew…you know, because it just takes your breath away. It feels like a shiver."

At this point, Jerry said, he's ready for the next phase. "Once I disconnect, I relax for a moment and review what I have seen. It seems this gift provides me a vivid photographic memory of all I saw. It's a scaleable memory, where I can go back to see the points that are lit up and examine those areas in greater detail if I need to."

Many people ask Jerry if he feels the person's pain. "Yes, this is usually part of my experience. But it isn't pain the way you experience pain in this realm. I can 'feel' it is painful, how intensely and where the pain is. It's a unique understanding of discomfort, but it doesn't interfere with the work I'm doing. It's a presence, I suppose, but it isn't the same kind of sensation as if I were to step on a tack."

In fact, for Jerry, the experience can be relaxing. "When I'm inside looking around," he says, "it's like I'm in that state, right in the middle of a good yawn, and if feels great. As I'm examining things, that feeling rises and falls ever so slightly."

Jerry has always believed the experience must be similar to a woman experiencing sexual pleasure. "I think a woman could understand it better than a man could. Because a woman in order to experience pleasure has to completely release. She has to allow and release. Whereas when a man experiences pleasure, it's almost like hold your breath and tense up. It's two totally different experiences. When I get to that point where I am ready to transfer healing energy, and it starts releasing, I can only imagine it must be very similar to that."

That's why Jerry says breathing is so important. "Because what you have to do is take that deep breath. It's almost like a sigh of relief moving through you. And within that moment you feel a total abandon of control. The feeling I have during that sigh moves through like a fire, but it doesn't feel burning like a fire would. When that moment comes, when I just allow and release this energy to move through, that's how it feels. It doesn't stop as long as I continue breathing. I'm so focused while this is happening that I'm not aware of anything out there around me."

And it isn't just pain Jerry feels. "If the person is using some pretty heavy duty drugs I will very likely be affected. For example, this little girl I worked on was pumped up with morphine. When I finished working with her, it was as though I was loaded with morphine. I couldn't walk. I could hardly talk. I had to be helped to a chair. I was just absolutely whacked on this stuff. I know that it's a passing thing, and within a short time I'll feel myself again. The reason I experience the effect is because the drugs have their own inherent energetic characteristics. They modify the electrical characteristics of the person using them. Once I merge with my client's energy field, the drugs modify mine as well. But the drugs, as a drug, aren't within me."

And for a healer, Jerry has an interesting way of dealing with the side effects of energy healing. He has a smoke. "The effects wear off very fast. If I have a cigarette, it fades away instantly. If I don't, it takes anywhere between fifteen minutes to a half hour to subside."

When Jerry pulls back and then begins to study what he's seen inside the client's body, he's looking for more than just one thing here or one thing there. He's looking for a connection. He finds that what's usually wrong with a person has to do with their energy flow. A problem in one part of the body may disrupt the flow of natural energy to another part.

"One place has a weakness, creating a weakness elsewhere," he said. "So I try to find that. I'm looking for that all the time. But when I finally digest the information and I make a comparison between what I've seen and the details they have provided me, their list and what they've said, I come to a conclusion about what is really going on, and why."

Jerry then moves his hands to the affected area. He found out long ago that he could best help someone if he actually touched the area he needed to heal. Again, he asks permission to touch his client first, and usually receives it.

This is when the healing begins, when Jerry uses his energy to find and then heal whatever is wrong.

The first time we discussed healing for this book, I asked Jerry, "How do you do it?"

"That's a good question," was Jerry's reply. Fortunately he expanded on his answer for me. "The way that I 'fix it', in simple terms, is that I dematerialize the areas that are injured. The item or area I'm working on becomes a parsed zone of energy within the quantum field I have created. Remember how I pull everything into me and that it manifests within me, but it is just energy? Well, the reverse is true as well. When I'm ready to correct or alter tissue, I determine what needs to be done. Next, I connect to the location I'm interested to work on and alter the area by parsing the energetic field. Isolating it this way allows me to work on a singular area without affecting, or being affected by, the surrounding tissue or otherwise the remainder of the body I am working within. Once this step is completed, I find the same area within my body. So far, there isn't really anything wrong with me, except for poor eyesight."

It's Jerry's own body – a healer's template if you will – that he will use to find differences, and therefore problems, with the client he's working on.

With his concentration now firmly fixed on healing his client, he sees into both his own body and that of the person he is working with. He uses his own energy flow to dematerialize the human tissue causing pain (for example) in his client's body. Then he rebuilds it, sometimes using his own body as a guide.

"Once it is in a vaporous state," he said, "it becomes soft and pliable. Then I use a template from the same area within myself to begin the healing process. For example, if I'm working on someone with a hip problem I might use the design from my hip to help this person's body know how to reconstruct their injured hip. I watch closely how the reformation is going and guide with minute detail if necessary. Though the process is actually a rapid one from the observer's perspective, I am moving my focus from one area to the next, just a little at a time, to reform, reshape and return the injured area to its normal shape and condition. The energy of this person's body wants it to be like that anyway in order for harmony to be restored to the body. So I provide that assistance. Using my body as a guide, I project this holographic template while tissue has been made so soft and pliable."

Jerry said complete healing isn't instantaneous – it takes time for the reshaped flesh and bones to become whole again. "By the time I'm finished, it's still soft. It hasn't finished 'cooking' yet. So, I tell them just to sit very still. At this stage it is important for them to relax, and keep breathing. I've closed the connection between myself and them to allow their body to stand on its own. Their field shifts and balances for a few minutes. I'll just leave it alone for a little bit. Once I notice their field has balanced I ask them to test the healing by moving or otherwise self observing how they feel. It's important to challenge the healing to find out if the process has been successful. This also provides my client an opportunity to realize intellectually the reality of the healing having taken place, and to what degree."

There are times, Jerry said, it might take more than one attempt to get it just right. "When I go back and check the area, and it's now solid enough where they can move, I ask them to put the healing to the test. Just because the tissue has been reformed doesn't mean that its reaction is going to be the same to movement as it ought to be. So I have them move. Sometimes I have them move with my fingertips around the area so I can watch all the intricacies. I can look at any angle in any area. If I see something is still wrong, I change it."

"The results are often instantly obvious," Jerry said. "About fifteen to twenty percent of the time restoration fades in, let's say, to where more and more benefits are received over time. I believe the reason that delay happens is simply because they can't get their minds around it. It can be very difficult to understand that one minute you were in pain and crippled up, and here you are the next minute and nothing is wrong – there is no pain and you can move as if nothing was ever wrong with you. Sometimes it doesn't register intellectually.

Rod Haberer

"That's why I have them push the situation." Jerry cites an example. A woman with a bad back had come to see him earlier that day. "She couldn't twist, she couldn't bend over. I finished, and said okay, twist, try to make it hurt, see what it takes to make it hurt. Like a lot of people I work with, she says it won't take much to make it hurt again. I say you're going to be surprised. Just do it, and if it hurts, I'll go back to work on it. In her case, as in the others, they twist this way, they twist that way. They timidly start bending over and up, and over and up, and finally they're doing deep knee squats. Then they put their palms on the floor, and they're just completely enthusiastic about how good they feel. This proves to them intellectually that something's happened. And those are the ones that really are astonishing, because then you can see in their eyes that they understand something has taken place that is beyond explanation."

For Jerry the experience is more than just rewarding. "I've just had an experience that's a very deep emotional and physical experience with them," he said. "And I feel really, really happy."

But what is energy healing? Where does he get the ability to do what he does? Those are obvious questions, but to Jerry, just as obviously difficult to answer. Because any answer would clearly alienate some people, while enthusiastically enriching others. Jerry says he knows exactly where his talents come from. "I'm absolutely certain, because I'm so familiar with it. I know how it works, I know why it works, and I know what it is and where it comes from. But I'm not sure if the general population is ready for this information or would understand if I explained it."

It's not just because he's judging our ability to comprehend. Jerry says it goes deeper than that. "It's only now that scientists are beginning to understand that things may not be as they seem. The universe is actually compiled as a result of our imagination. We are not the result of the universe's existence. The universe is the result of our presence."

"The presence of this energy, the creative force, has from ancient times been called many things," Jerry said. "And it's been called God. During the last two thousand years God has always been portrayed as a figure. It is remarkably difficult to fear, respect or obey divine direction without a figure in place to direct your attention. In reality, God is within every form, but is none of them."

What Jerry is talking about is a life force. "This force," he said, "is an energetic presence always ready, willing and able to become creative force. It's what everything springs from and goes back to. It starts within us and moves outward. It is beyond our comprehension yet moves toward and into us as if we and it know each other well. We're part of a larger thing, and are that larger thing, all at the same time."

Does this sound familiar? I asked Jerry if "The Force" portrayed in the story of a Galaxy far, far away called <u>Star Wars</u> is similar.

"Yes, in many ways we're talking about a similar understanding," he admitted. "The philosophical concepts illustrated in <u>Star Wars</u>, like the Jedi, are based upon Eastern principles. For example, the instruction Luke received from Yoda. The implementation of the teaching was turned into a hard to believe cartoon-like thing in the movie. But when you consider what Yoda was trying to do with Luke Skywalker, you can only arrive to one conclusion. He told him to have confidence. Raise the ship out of the mud. Compare that to scientific documentation of what one group of monks in Pakistan can do. They get together once every year and sit in front of this boulder that weighs several tons, and start chanting. They raise the boulder up into the air and then slowly set it back down again. So I believe there are elements of reality within <u>Star Wars</u>. It's just that you have to be open minded enough to consider these unique and available possibilities."

When most people ask Jerry where his powers come from, he has a more direct response. "I just tell them it's the presence of the Divine, the Creator... it's God."

To Jerry, it's all the same thing. "When we speak about this force that moves through me as I work on someone, it's easy to attribute this to being a unique and singular ability I have that others have no access to. This is not the case at all. What I am accessing is the same force moving through everyone. It's always there and always available. The greatest difference between me and another who is trying to access it is that I've developed my skill over time by being curious and staying aware. I've figured out how to play with it, how to use it constructively."

And guess what? There is a dark side to this force. Jerry's seen it. "This force can also be used in a destructive way. The same thing that can cause a person's back to heal instantly can also be used in just the opposite way. It all stems from intention, desire and an emotional connection to what you're doing. My intention is to help in whatever way I can to ease pain, to bring hope and to give them light, and most of all to give my clients a reason to see beyond their current situation."

As for non-believers—Jerry says it really doesn't matter if you believe or not. "It doesn't matter," he says. "I have no idea what a person's belief is when they are unconscious or in a coma. What's the belief structure of a child?" he asked. "It really doesn't matter if a person believes or not."

"What matters the most," Jerry says, "is what I believe."

For Jerry, the moment when he sees someone finally free of pain or their Infirmity is the happiest he ever feels. "I just feel very, very at peace, like everything is right with the world," he said. "It's one of those feelings like there's nothing that's bothering me. You just feel completely safe, you feel okay and everything is right with the world."

The healer has done his job.

As Jerry's client base grows, so does a long list of people who believe there is something special in the world. And they believe that maybe Jerry is a very special person.

The facts of Jerry's past, present, and future are sometimes tragic, sometimes mysterious, but always amazing. What is clear is that he didn't reach this point by accident. He's helping others now because he believes that is why he's been put on this Earth. Not to make millions of dollars entertaining and healing for profit. He's here to bring awareness of something that's been missing in many of our lives.

In this introduction, I've tried to provide you the reader with a brief glimpse into what is possible. In the following pages you will learn how Jerry reached this point. You will read about his awakening after a tragic near-death experience. You will hear from others he has helped. You will also find out how the mysteries of South America have led Jerry on a path of discovery that is very much a part of his being.

And finally, you will learn how Jerry is passing his abilities on to others. Because Jerry believes he was put on this Earth not to just help others – but to help others help themselves. Jerry and many others believe we are at a crossroads; one age is coming to an end and another one is beginning. Those who cross from one to the other will need to believe in more than just the New York Stock Exchange, and they will need to be armed with more than a gun. The changing times will come at a price – but the benefit will be mankind's survival. Jerry believes he is here to help us cross over. Only time will tell if he is right.

I'm still a skeptic by training and by nature. I can't prove what Jerry does works, even after talking to dozens of people who believe Jerry cured them. I can't disprove it either. In fact, I would challenge anyone out there to prove it to me one way or the other. All I know is that most of the people Jerry works on are suddenly better. Their pain is gone. Was it Western medicine that cured them, or the energy that Jerry used to manipulate and destroy whatever ailed them? I don't know. Was it a combination of the two? Still, I don't know. Once again, read the book and make up your own mind.

So, let's start our journey down the rabbit hole. I hope you enjoy the ride.

Chapter One
Born in Kentucky?

He's just a baby…and he's flying.

The child is only a few months old. He doesn't even have a name yet; he doesn't know where he is. But he does know he is being held in a woman's arms, and he is being loved. Feelings of warmth and happiness fill his soul, and his heart is light and happy.

He glances out what seems to be a large window. They are in some sort of aircraft flying across the treetops. The window is bubble-shaped and clear, and they are moving fast and very low over trees and open fields. It seems to the boy as if some of the taller trees might reach out to touch them.

As the woman holding him sings him a lullaby in a language he doesn't understand, the child who will become Jerry Wills thinks the song is beautiful, and somehow the words make perfect sense. As he listens to the lullaby Jerry feels movement, and continues to watch the treetops slip below him. But it's warm and cozy in the woman's arms, and she smells good. Jerry feels very safe.

He also sees two moons in the night sky, at least he thinks they are moons. He really doesn't know what they are. They seem to glide over the treetops with them, silent glowing orbs that follow their every move like bright shadows against the dark but starlit sky.

Then the ride is over. They slowly come to a stop, and settle to the ground below. A man joins them. Jerry doesn't know who he is, but he escorts Jerry and the woman holding him out of the aircraft and into some sort of small building. It's empty, and smells musty. There is no furniture, so the woman spreads a blanket on the ground and sets Jerry on the blanket. It's cold and dark, Jerry is shivering. So the woman puts another blanket around Jerry. The small boy looks up at the woman and man with a quizzical look. They look down on him, and she seems to have a very sad expression on her face. She also stopped singing. Then she bends down and gives Jerry a kiss on the top of his head. Jerry tries to reach up through the blankets with his small arms, but the woman does not pick him up. She says something, very softly, that Jerry doesn't understand. Then she and the man turn their backs and walk away.

Jerry is left there, all alone. He waits for them to come back, but they never do. He's in a vacant building, maybe an old home, somewhere in the countryside. It's 1953. But Jerry really doesn't know what year it is, or where he is. He only knows that he's alone. As the blanket slips from his shoulders, he begins to shiver again. He's cold and frightened, but most of all curious about why he was left there, and why the woman won't come back.

After what seems like several hours later, Jerry notices a loud noise outside. Maybe they've come back. But the boy soon realizes it's not the woman. There's a very loud noise as helicopters hover overhead, and several Jeeps and trucks pull up outside, their bright headlights shining through the broken windows, temporarily blinding Jerry. Several men in uniform carrying rifles come running into the building. They surround Jerry and look down at him. Another man walks up to him, bends down and picks him up. He is wearing what looks to Jerry like a funny, large, flat hat. Jerry was later told that they were from the U.S. Army Air Corps, from a military base near the empty home.

Soon Jerry is in the back of a truck, still being held by the man with a funny hat. Another man is looking at Jerry, holding his arm, and shining a light in his eyes. They soon arrive at some sort of hospital with lots of men in white coats staring down at him. He doesn't know where he is yet, but it turns out Jerry is a guest at the U.S. Army's Fort Knox, Kentucky.

Why Fort Knox? Why Kentucky? Jerry doesn't really know, and he's never told. He only knows what his birth certificate says. It says Jerry was born on September 11th, 1953, at Fort Knox, Kentucky (See the photo section of this book for a copy of Jerry's birth certificate). Jerry lived at the base hospital for some time, but soon a man and woman came to the hospital and took him home. They were kind and loving, but not the same two people who left Jerry alone that night not so long ago. But he would come to accept the man and woman who took him home as his parents.

They never told young Jerry that he was adopted. To Jerry at the time, they were just Mom and Dad.

Jerry's father's name was Dwight Wills. He usually wore an Army uniform, but Jerry didn't know what he did. His friends called him Ace. His mother's name was MaeBelle Wills; her maiden name was Church.

Shortly after they took Jerry from the base hospital, the Wills family moved to Denver, Colorado. Jerry was told that his father had a government job, and his new job was in Denver. He never found out what his father really did for the government, but he made enough money for the three of them to live comfortably in a small home just outside town. Jerry liked it in Denver. He liked to play in the snow with his mom, and he liked school.

Jerry had a normal childhood in Denver, for the most part. The only times he would get in trouble was if he would write with both hands or try to help someone. If a person came to visit his mother or Ace and that person was sick or injured, Jerry wanted to touch that person instinctively. He knew he could make them better. But he was usually scolded and told it was not polite to touch people.

Jerry also liked the yearly trips he took to Florida with his dad. His father always said they were going to Florida to visit Jerry's "uncle."

By the time he was five-years-old, the trips to Florida started to seem strange to Jerry because neither his mother nor father had any family who lived in Florida. Jerry really didn't know who this uncle was. He only knew that once every year they would visit Florida. His uncle would pick them up in a big, black Cadillac sedan and drive Jerry and his father along a highway for several hours.

Each time they would drive into the wilderness of Florida's Everglades. To a young Jerry, it was a huge, mysterious but exciting place. Jerry imagined all kinds of creatures hiding behind the huge trees and thick undergrowth of the Florida swamp. In some places, the trees and brush were so thick, they blocked out the sun. Jerry could only see a few feet into the forest itself. But like any five-year-old, Jerry wondered what it would be like to explore the dense, swampy forest.

He also noticed there were no buildings, no signs, no light posts for miles on end.

With his uncle driving, Jerry and his father sat mostly silent, staring out the windows. His mother was left behind. She never came along on one of Jerry's special trips.

Eventually, they pulled off the highway onto a dirt road and drove down it for quite a while, bounding along, going fast as hell. Jerry bounced up and down on the seat as they went. It was fun.

Jerry also liked looking at his uncle's gun. It was in a holster, and Jerry imagined he was some kind of cop or sheriff, maybe. He never asked.

Finally, they pulled up to a gate and stopped the car. The gate had a sign on it that said U.S. Government, No Trespassing.

"Hey, Dad, the sign says we can't go in there," Jerry said. At five-years-old, Jerry could already read.

"Don't worry, son," his father said, "We have permission. It's fine. Your Uncle Sam owns this and it's okay with him, so if it's okay with him, we can go in."

"Okay, Dad," Jerry said, just happy that his adventure would continue.

They left the car and walked into the area on foot. Eventually they came to a place where a small rowboat was tied up.

"Cool," Jerry said. "Can we take a boat ride?"

"We sure can, Jerry," his father said. "Jump in."

Jerry hopped right into the boat first. His father and uncle were right behind him. The boat had a small motor, but to Jerry's dismay they didn't use it. Instead Jerry's father and the man Jerry thought of as Uncle Sam used paddles to slowly move them down a small stream. Jerry thought it would be cooler if they used the motor to go fast…but instead, slowly and silently they rowed. Again, the two men said nothing while Jerry peered into the Everglades from his seat at the bow of the small boat.

Jerry couldn't tell where they were heading. All he could see was the swamp and heavy forest all around him. The water they were moving through had a greenish tint to it, and every once in a while he would see a pool full of greenish, stagnant water. It smelled funny, too.

Finally they rowed toward what looked like a very large stand of trees. But they still rowed silently along a stream that wove itself in and out of the forest all around them. Jerry watched his father swat a mosquito that looked like a small bird. It was huge. Jerry checked the back of his neck to make sure there wasn't one on him.

The swamp was also a very loud place. Jerry could hear all kinds of things he couldn't begin to identify. He did see some frogs, a lot more bugs, and maybe a glimpse of a small snake. To Jerry, the whole place seemed alive. At one point Jerry was beginning to wonder how far they had come. He had lost himself paying attention to all the life buzzing about him.

Then something even more curious got his attention. His father and uncle stopped rowing as they approached what looked like a huge wall covered with weeds and moss. His uncle raised one of the paddles, and banged it on the wall…

Bang, bang, bang! "That should wake them up," his Uncle Sam said.

"They're already here," Jerry's father replied.

"Who is?" Jerry asked.

"Just watch," was all his father would say.ry sat there, mystified, and a bit bored. But then he saw two men show up. At least he thought they were men. They were covered in what looked like weeds. Jerry could barely see them, only after they moved. He thought it very weird, and was a little frightened.

"Wow," Jerry said. "Dad, are they all right?"

"Yes," his father said. "Don't worry, they're with us." He smiled down at his son. "Pretty amazing, huh? They were here all along."

Jerry watched in amazement as the two men pulled some ropes, and the wall of weeds lifted over them like a garage door. Jerry's father and his uncle continued to row the boat as they went underneath the now removable wall. Jerry saw real vines clinging to the wall as they slowly moved under it. He smiled broadly, and thought it was the coolest thing he had ever seen.

Soon they were out of the boat and walking along a dirt path. The men wearing "weeds", what Jerry would know later as camouflage, accompanied them. Sometimes they were right next to them. At other times Jerry could see one moving in the distance. Of course, like any boy, Jerry was fascinated with the guns and knives these men carried with them.

It took a while, but eventually Jerry could see something that looked like a small camp. There was a large grassy area where the swamp and forest had been pushed back. There were some buildings that were at least partially made of canvas. It was nothing that looked very permanent, more tent-like. Some men came out to greet them, and they talked quietly with Jerry's father and uncle.

Shortly some more men appeared, and these really caught Jerry's attention. They wore clean white outfits, like a doctor or nurse in a hospital would wear. But some of them had on space suits, at least what Jerry thought of as space suits, with helmets and gloves.

One of them walked up to Jerry. He looked at his father, who said, "It's okay, Jerry. Don't be afraid. He's not going to hurt you."

One of the soldiers Jerry had seen during previous visits here held out a pack of gum in his right hand. "Hi there, Jerry," he said. "Want a stick of gum?"

Jerry just nodded yes, not sure what to say. He quickly grabbed a stick of gum from the pack in the man's hand, and took a couple of steps back.

"Thank you," was all he could manage.

Jerry looked down at the stick of Juicy-Fruit gum in his hands, and he unwrapped it.

The man who gave him the gum said, "It's nice to see you again, Jerry. How have you been doing?"

"Fine, Sir, "Jerry said. "Thanks again for the gum."

"You are welcome."

Jerry recognized a military insignia on the man's uniform, so he knew he was in the military like his dad. That always provided some comfort. He also carried a gun, a rifle slung on his shoulder. He was also always smoking a cigarette.

Jerry popped the gum in his mouth, and smiled. He liked Juicy-Fruit.

With his father and uncle looking on, Jerry was escorted into one of the larger tents in the camp.

More men in white outfits and space helmets were inside the tent, and all of them were looking at Jerry.

The next thing Jerry knows, he's waking up back in a hotel room with his mother and father. "Good morning, Sunshine," his mother said. "Time to get up, we're going to the beach this morning."

"Mom, Dad, what happened? Where are all the guys in white?" Jerry asked.

"Oh, they're gone, Jerry," his father said. "Try not to think about it. We're going to the beach to have some fun."

"Okay," Jerry said. It happened year after year, for at least six years straight. Jerry just began to think of it as normal. He must have fallen asleep or something. He really didn't worry about it all that much. Besides, they were going to the beach, and Jerry loved it there.

Later that same year, Jerry's father took him to a Masonic Temple in Denver. After getting out of the car, Jerry and his father walked around a large building and went in the backdoor. After Jerry's father showed another man his identification, which Jerry thought was very cool, the two of them went down a narrow stairway.

Then they took an elevator and went down even further. Jerry wondered how far they were going. "Dad, where does this elevator go?" he asked.

"Just down to another room. We're going to meet some people, so be on your best behavior, Jerry."

"Okay." Jerry was happy to be on another adventure with his dad. He liked going out with him.

Eventually, the elevator opened to a big room, and it was full of people. Most of them were talking in hushed tones. Jerry was having a hard time making out what they were saying, and he thought that was strange.

Soon, an older man came up to Jerry's father, and asked if he could introduce himself to Jerry. "I must meet this young man," he said, and he reached out to shake Jerry's hand.

Jerry looked up at his father.

"It's all right, Jerry," he said. "These people all want to meet you."

"Hello there, Jerry," the man said still holding out his hand. "I'm Mr. Peters, a friend of your father."

Jerry took his hand and shook it.

"Nice to meet you, Sir," Jerry said.

The man smiled back, and said, "It's nice to meet you. What a gentleman," he said smiling at Jerry's father.

Jerry's father smiled, too, and gently patted his son's back.

On and on it went for some time. Jerry's father stood there next to his son as man after man came up to meet Jerry. They never said much; they only said they wanted to meet Ace's "son."

Jerry really didn't understand what it was all about. No one ever explained anything to him. He also met other people who mentioned they were with the government. Some said they were senators; others were congressmen. They all seemed to know his father very well. In fact, they seemed to know more about Jerry's dad than Jerry did.

Jerry had turned seven in September, and his father died in December of that same year. Jerry doesn't know what killed him. At this point, Jerry still thought of them as his real mother and father. He would only find out later that Dwight Wills and MaeBelle Wills were incapable of having children.

The next year, Jerry and his mother moved back to Kentucky where MaeBelle had family. But only after a new scare in Denver. After his father died, some men came to the door. They wanted to take Jerry away, but his mother wouldn't let them.

"You will not take my son, and you will leave us alone!" she yelled at the men standing in the door. "Jerry is my son; he's legally adopted. You can't do anything about it." She then slammed the door in their faces.

"Mom, why do they want to take me?" Jerry asked.

"Don't you worry about them," she said. "They won't bother us any longer. Besides, we're moving."

"Okay," Jerry said. Moving sounded like a lot of fun. But he had another question. "What's adopted mean?" he asked.

His mother hadn't intended for Jerry to overhear her yelling match with the men at the door. "Don't you worry about it," she said. "You are my son, and there will be no more talk of you going with anyone."

"Okay, Mom," Jerry said. He would later figure out on his own what adopted meant, but he wouldn't ask his mother about it again.

The next day, MaeBelle Wills packed their bags, and drove herself and Jerry from Denver to Kentucky. They soon moved in with her sister.

Jerry's Aunt Louise lived in Elizabethtown, Kentucky, where he and his mother lived for a time.

13

Her home wasn't big enough for them, so they worked for a few weeks to fix up a chicken coup on the side of a hill. Eventually they turned it into a one-room house with a kitchen on one side, the bed on the other. The hill was steep, and Jerry had to be careful just walking out the front door. After about four feet, the hill dropped away into a near vertical fall. It was farm property, but Jerry's Aunt Louise and her husband Joe didn't do any farming. It was about thirty acres, so Jerry had plenty of space to explore.

They also spent time with Jerry's grandmother (At least with the person Jerry thought of as his grandmother – the two were actually not related). Her home was near a little town called Eighty-Eight in Kentucky. The town was on Highway 88, hence the name. It consisted of a store and a post office, both in the same building. That was it.

Jerry heard that his grandmother had a special gift, that if someone were hurt, she could heal them. But it scared many people who lived in the area, so she never really used it. Jerry had never actually seen his grandmother heal anybody; to him it was just a story.

One day Jerry's mother dropped him off to spend the weekend with his grandmother while she looked for work. The home seemed to be in the middle of nowhere, surrounded by thick stands of trees, and lots of wild undergrowth.

There was a big hill outside, perfect for rolling. So, that's what Jerry did-- he rolled downhill, got up, brushed off the grass and plants sticking to him, climbed back up the hill and did it again.

His grandmother saw him and was immediately concerned. "Jerry," she yelled from the front porch of the house, "that's poison ivy you're rolling in! Come up here!"

Jerry walked up to his grandmother, and she looked him over. "You're going to be in one world of hurt, boy." She was really worried. She didn't want to turn Jerry back over to his mother covered in a skin rash.

"Don't worry, Grandma," Jerry said, "I'll be okay."

"Sure," she said, "you say that now, but just you wait." His grandmother started wiping the sticks, dirt and the poison ivy off him. It was everywhere.

Suddenly she stopped, and gave Jerry a funny look. Then she gasped, and said, "Oh my God, Child. You've got the gift."

"What's the gift?" Jerry asked.

"You'll never have anything wrong with you. You don't get sick, do you, child?"

"No, I don't."

"I just wish I knew where they got you. You are one special child, Jerry." His grandmother seemed all aflutter and excited.

She took Jerry back into the house and made him some hot chocolate.

From that point forward, she never showed Jerry much of anything. But, "she told me that I always had to be aware that people would be watching. That if I figured out how to use this gift, then I'm likely to frighten people. I never asked her any details of her gift. I figured she just had it."

His grandmother had black hair with a white streak running through it. And Jerry would always remember her as the nicest person he'd ever met. She also made him the best oatmeal he ever had.

Jerry and his mother lived in her sister's one-room chicken coup home for about a year. Then they moved to another house farther from town. Soon they moved again, and again. In the meantime, MaeBelle remarried. Eventually their family added Jerry's two sisters, Lynn and Lori, who only recently discovered they might have been adopted. Jerry didn't get along with his stepdad. "He was cruel and insensitive, not very well educated, and not very nice to me from the very beginning."

Jerry's stepdad was an alcoholic, and not very nice to his mother either, something that really bothered Jerry. But there wasn't much he could do about it. Jerry spent most of his time at school, or exploring the countryside, trying to stay as far away from his stepdad as he could. He was afraid of him. But the experience helped-- and hurt-- Jerry. "I learned that being afraid of someone is not a state of being to remain in for long. My sisters were the focus of the family, I was just an added feature. They thought of me as someone who could work around the farm. I didn't like that much."

But soon, Jerry would discover something he liked doing. It all started with a mouse.

Chapter Two
The Healer Within

He was twelve-years-old, living on another farm in Kentucky. Jerry Wills liked to wander about the place while doing his best to avoid his stepfather.

Jerry was spending more time with animals than he was with the rest of his family. He liked the peace they brought him and he found them restful. Soon, young Jerry found he could communicate with animals on the farm and in the nearby wooded areas in that part of Kentucky. He thought it was great. Jerry couldn't actually talk with them but he could sense what they were feeling and communicate by different forms of imagery he could share with them.

Jerry would whistle to the birds, and they would whistle back. They would fly around and land near him unafraid. In fact, none of the animals who lived on the farm or nearby seemed afraid of Jerry, and he liked being part of their world.

One day Jerry was in an old shed on the farm and he saw one of the mice he had been communicating with. It was dead, the victim of a mousetrap.

It was a cold November day with snow already on the ground. Jerry was horrified when he saw the crushed mouse in the trap so he stopped what he was doing and reached down to pick up the dead mouse. He had to work to push back the strong spring, holding the trap in place with his thumb while he removed the mouse with his left hand. He carefully removed his thumb from the trap and threw the now empty trap into the snow.

Jerry looked at the dead mouse in his hand, thinking that it just wasn't right to kill a mouse that way. It seemed cruel. It seemed an awful thing to do to a living creature.

After first glancing behind him to make sure no one was there, Jerry put the mouse in his right hand and put his left hand over it. He thought if he warmed it up a bit maybe the mouse would be all right. He breathed into his hand, hoping to keep the mouse warm. He just kept breathing on it. Four or five times he took deep breaths and exhaled into his hands.

Then, to his surprise, Jerry felt movement in his hand. Jerry breathed on it one more time and lifted his left hand to take a peak. There looking at him was the mouse, looking like a mouse should look. Its ears were perked up and he was looking at Jerry. Jerry laughed as its nose wiggled back and forth and as the mouse looked at Jerry inquisitively.

Jerry said to himself, "Wow, that's pretty cool. You're alive."

The mouse just stood there in Jerry's hand looking at him.

Jerry didn't want to see the mouse in that trap again, so he gave the mouse a good talking to.

By showing the mouse what the traps could do in his mind, Jerry told the mouse not to go anywhere near the things. And the mouse seemed to be paying attention. After all, just a few moments before the mouse had been dead.

Jerry then received a message from the mouse. He saw a picture in his mind of the mouse and his children. Apparently, the mouse was trying to get them food. Jerry also realized that the mouse he had just saved was the father and it struck Jerry as strange that it was a male mouse. He never considered a mouse being male or female before; it just never occurred to him. Having babies never occurred to him either.

Jerry showed the mouse images of Jerry leaving food for him and his family under the floorboards of the shed. The shed had some old boards on the floor and snow would blow through them. It had a foundation board around the outside, and the floor was suspended a good foot or so above the ground. Jerry showed the mouse that he would drop food down through the cracks in the floor, as much as the mouse needed. And he again warned the mouse that when he came looking for food to stay away from the traps. He also told the mouse to tell his babies the same thing.

Jerry demonstrated to the mouse he would make sure they had plenty of food, especially during the winter. The mouse could also tell all his friends if they needed more food to just to let him know and there will be plenty for everyone.

21

After that day, Jerry would take food meant for the farm's cows...they had plenty anyway...and delivered it to the mice on a regular basis. His stepfather never caught another mouse in one of his mouse traps, and he always wondered why the traps never worked.

Besides mice and cows, Jerry's family farm also had some pigs, but they didn't last very long. After all, it was a farm and there was nothing Jerry could do about that. Most of the cows were milk cows so they got to stay. Jerry was up at five-thirty every morning to feed the cows and pigs. Dropping some food for the mice took no time at all.

After feeding the animals, Jerry would chop some wood for the wood stove in the house then head off for school.

The cold Kentucky winters really bothered Jerry a lot. He never had shoes that fit right, and his feet were always cold. He was always fighting frostbite.

His parents eventually discovered the Army surplus store, and they bought clothes and boots for Jerry there. He had plenty of Army surplus clothes and was always wearing fatigues and boots to school. Jerry was growing so fast, it was the only way his family could afford to keep him in shoes and clothes that fit. He quickly outgrew several new pairs of boots every year.

But it was also an enchanting time for Jerry. When he wasn't worried about staying warm, he would be outside communicating with animals. He felt as if talking to people was a waste of time. Jerry could already read instinctively what was in their head; he could feel what was in their heart and he knew what was going on. Most of the time he didn't like the feelings he got looking into the minds of people, so over time it was something he learned to block out.

Animals were different. They were pure. They were either hungry or they were not. They were either happy or they were not.

Jerry found that birds didn't have any reason to be unhappy. They would get excited when a cat was around but he never found unhappy birds. They were just curious.

Cows were always introverted and not easy to strike up a conversation with. Jerry found that dogs were mostly goofy. They just wanted to play. Jerry found foxes very interesting because they would look at him and think that Jerry could not see them. Jerry would communicate back of course that he could see them just fine. The foxes didn't like that very much.

Ground hogs and squirrels around the farm were often communicating with Jerry as well, again by telepathic imagery. They were always looking for food.

As for the people Jerry talked to, most of them found him odd. One day the town preacher told Jerry's mother and stepfather that it was time for Jerry to be baptized. Jerry was thirteen at the time, and they dunked him into a stream of water. Jerry found it to be an awful experience.

"You can't go to heaven if you don't get baptized, Jerry," his mother said.

Give me a break, thought Jerry to himself. Why would he want to stop the journey now?

It was later that summer that the same preacher decided it would be good if he took Jerry squirrel hunting. Jerry was horrified. He'd already been back in the woods talking to the squirrels; they were his friends. He was worried, and he didn't want to go. But Jerry thought that if he didn't go on the hunting trip, the preacher might shoot one. He decided to go and figure out a way to warn them.

The preacher gave Jerry a .22-caliber rifle, and off into the woods they went.

"We'll head to a spot where I know there are plenty of squirrels," the preacher said.

"Why do you want to shoot one?" Jerry asked.

"Jerry," the Preacher said, "God put these animals on Earth for us to use, to survive. We hunt them and eat them to celebrate His power on Earth."

To Jerry, that made no sense at all.

They continued walking back into the woods, and to Jerry's horror, they hiked to the exact spot where Jerry liked to go to be alone, and talk to his friends. But now it was going to be a killing ground.

The preacher told Jerry to have a seat on a nearby stump, and he started telling Jerry about God and Jesus, and how to open his heart to them and the church. All the time, Jerry is just thinking about how in the world he is going to save the squirrels he knows.

"The small animals in this forest, Jerry," the preacher said, "God put on this Earth for us to use. So, it's okay to hunt them if it's God's will."

Jerry was still unconvinced. "What do you think the animals would say?" Jerry asked the preacher.

"Jerry," the Preacher said, "they're just dumb animals, son. They can't communicate."

"That's not true," Jerry said. "And I can prove it."

"Don't be ridiculous," The preacher said. "Look, there's a squirrel now."

Jerry watched as the preacher aimed his weapon at the animal Jerry had communicated with many times before.

"Can I shoot it?" Jerry asked the preacher.

The man was startled by Jerry's sudden request. He lowered his weapon and said, "Sure, go ahead. He's all yours."

Jerry knew it was a female squirrel, but didn't bother correcting the preacher. Instead he took aim, and fired, but nowhere near the squirrel. The shot went ricocheting off a tree and all the squirrels took off running. Of course, it was exactly as Jerry intended.

He didn't stop there. Jerry kept shooting all over the place. Bullets were bouncing off rocks and trees – every squirrel within a half mile scurried away. He kept firing until the rifle was out of bullets.

"I think I missed," Jerry told the preacher.

"Missed? Of course you missed. Why did you do that? You scared them all away." The preacher was obviously missing the point.

"You're exactly right, Sir," Jerry said, clearing it up for him. "I did exactly that. These squirrels are my friends. Why would I want to kill them? Why do you want to kill them? You're a preacher."

Jerry threw down the rifle and walked home.

The preacher was pretty upset with Jerry, and he told his stepfather all about it. Jerry's stepfather, Elmer, threatened to beat Jerry for being so obnoxious to the preacher, but Jerry showed no regret.

"Those squirrels are alive today, thanks to me," he told his stepfather. Jerry felt great, and he never regretted doing it.

A similar incident happened on a deer hunt Jerry found out about. Jerry was fifteen-years-old at the time.

He didn't know the deer; he never got around to visiting with them. But he always saw them in the distance. He took a handful of firecrackers with him, the kind that are all strung together. He followed the hunters out into the forest, and as soon as he saw them set up a blind to shoot the deer from, Jerry climbed up in an old oak tree just off to the side.

When Jerry saw the deer moving toward them, he lit the string of firecrackers and threw them near the deer. The firecrackers scared the deer off, and angered the hunters.

"There will be no deer hunting today," Jerry announced as he climbed down the tree.

The hunters swore at him, called him all kinds of names. Jerry didn't care. He stood there with a big smile on his face until the hunters started walking home.

Jerry was known mostly as a loner. By the time he was in high school, he had only two friends. Their first names were David and Randy. Most others found Jerry odd because he was usually dressed in Army surplus clothing.

Jerry had very, very short hair, and he was always alone. He was also a book worm, with a memory that allowed him to read something once and never forget it. He could also read very fast, and not even a comma would escape him. Request a quote from any book he had read, and Jerry could tell you the page number and every detail about that page. Some said he had a photographic memory.

The school Jerry attended gave him an IQ test, but it was discarded because Jerry's score was too high. They thought he cheated. So the next time, they made him sit at a desk and had at least one person watch him at all times. After he took the test a second, and then a third time, he got tired of it. The next time, Jerry answered a lot of questions wrong on purpose.

His guidance counselor knew what was happening. "Jerry, why didn't you do your best on that last test?" he asked.

"The test is stupid," Jerry said. "And I'm tired of taking them. I don't want to take any more tests."

Because Jerry was already very tall – he was six feet, seven inches as a high school sophomore – Jerry was told he needed to play on the basketball team, so he did. Most of the guys on the team had been playing basketball for years. Jerry had never played before. They didn't like him much because the only reason he was on the team was his height.

While playing basketball, he discovered he could help some of his teammates the same way he helped the mouse. If one of them twisted or sprained an ankle, Jerry would ask if he could take a look.

"Can I see that?" Jerry asked one player who sprained an ankle.

"What are you, a doctor or something?"

"No," Jerry responded, "I just wanted to take a look."

"Okay," the player said, wincing in pain as he raised his ankle so Jerry could hold it.

A few seconds later, the pain was gone. The player was startled – looking wide eyed at Jerry. "How did you do that?"

"Oh, it's nothing," Jerry said as he took a seat back on the bench.

After that, the players looked at Jerry funny, and he didn't like it. So from then on, Jerry did his healing in secret, never talking to his teammates. He discovered if he concentrated enough he could see their injuries without even touching them.

Off the basketball court, Jerry continued to spend most of his free time on the farm, with the animals. One day one of his dogs was shot. Part of his right hip was torn away by a shotgun blast. Jerry remembered what he had done for the mouse and wondered if he could help the dog.

The wound was just the most awful thing he'd ever seen. At first, he wasn't sure what to do. So he asked his stepfather about it.

Of course, he didn't care. "Leave it alone," his stepfather said. "Let him go off and die, it's what dogs do."

Jerry thought that wasn't right. The dog had to be hurting. He had to do something.

Jerry went down to a nearby creek and got a bucketful of mud. He put his hands in it and moved it around a bit, adding some water so it had the right consistency. How did he know it was the right consistency? He didn't, but after mixing in some mud it just seemed right.

The dog was trying to stand but couldn't. Jerry could clearly see and feel the panic and pain it felt.

"Calm down, boy," Jerry said as he slowly approached the dog. He sent the animal a mental picture of calmness. The dog stopped trying to get up, and lay down so Jerry could approach him. Jerry slowly spread his mud over the wound as the dog lay quietly. The wound still looked awful, and it smelled funny, but the mud seemed to help. Then Jerry placed his hand on the wound and tried his best to take away the pain.

When he finished, Jerry again communicated with the dog, encouraging it to fall asleep. The dog immediately nodded off.

The very next day, Jerry saw that his dog was up and walking, still limping quite a bit, but obviously better. The mud patch on his hind leg was still there. The patch seemed to be holding, and his dog was clearly doing better. The dog was never the same again, but the wound healed. The combination of mud and Jerry's healing abilities saved the dog from a certain, painful death. Jerry wasn't sure what he had done, but he knew he made a difference.

One day, Jerry noticed one of the cows was in pain. Jerry walked over and put his hands on the cow's hips. Normally, they would run away if a person approached, but not this time. Again, Jerry was able to calm the animal by communicating a peaceful scene. But maybe, thought Jerry, it didn't run away because it was hurting.

Jerry held his hands on the cow's hips and this time, Jerry felt his hands get really hot. For the first time as well, Jerry could also see the problem in his mind. The cow had a dislocated hip. When he finished putting the hip back into place and remolding the soft tissue around the joint to strengthen it, the cow just sort of walked away. It was never in pain again.

His first healing experiences with animals did not seem as amazing to Jerry as they might have to others. Jerry thought it was just a natural thing to do. Like it had when he was just a little boy, healing came to him instinctively.

Besides working on a few sprained ankles, Jerry's first major healing effort on a human being was when he tried to help a neighboring farmer.

The man couldn't walk because he had hurt his knee. He was in a lot of pain.

Jerry and the man were sharing some watermelon on a hot summer afternoon. Jerry liked him, because unlike his stepfather, the farmer was someone he could talk to.

"How is your knee?" Jerry asked.

"I'm in a lot of pain. It's not good," the farmer answered.

"Can I take a look at it?" Jerry asked.

"Why?"

"Maybe I can help." Jerry reached over, and just tapped the man's knee a couple of times. "Does that feel better?" he asked.

The farmer rose and flexed his knee a couple of times. Then he took a few steps. "I think it did, ah, it feels better. How did you do that?"

"Oh, it's nothing," said Jerry who went back to eating his watermelon as the farmer stared at him. Like his experience with the basketball player, the experience frightened the farmer who from then on looked at Jerry differently. Jerry wouldn't do that again.

As time went on, working on people became more and more difficult for Jerry. Because of the early reactions he received as a child and then as a teenager, he developed an aversion for touching people. He didn't want that kind of contact, and he didn't want to put his hands on another person at all. Despite what his instincts were telling him, his feelings now told him to stay away from other people.

The most profound event to shape Jerry's view of the world and living energy happened not with people or animals, but with a weed.

Jerry had just finished a book by Ruth Montgomery called Here and Hereafter. The book was all about a number of psychic events and past life experiences. Jerry found it very interesting.

Jerry put down the book, remembering his stepfather had ordered him to pull the weeds in a small family vegetable garden. It was late in the day, with the sun nearly setting behind some hills when Jerry grabbed a hoe and went to work on the weeds.

As Jerry chopped at the weeds in the fading light, he saw sparks. Thinking he was striking some rocks with the hoe blade, he continued on. But every time he carefully chopped a weed he would see a small spark. So he got down on the ground to take a closer look.

Kneeling in the dirt on that late afternoon, what Jerry saw first startled, and then amazed him. He could see a faint light coming from the very place where the weed stem was broken by the hoe. To Jerry it was evidence of life, of pain, and of a life force he was just beginning to comprehend.

After that, he spent more time in the garden, carefully watching weeds grow.

"What are you doing?" his stepfather asked once. "I said pull those weeds. Don't just sit there looking at them like an idiot."

From then on it bothered Jerry to pull or cut up weeds, because this was his first experience viewing the life force from a living organism. The longer he sat and watched it, the more detail he could see. He could take his fingers and move them into the light, and the light would move toward him. He could feel it tugging toward his fingers like it wanted to connect with him. It was a very spiritual experience and an awakening for young Jerry Wills. Here was life - he could see it and he could touch it. It was truly amazing.

One day when his stepfather was sleeping, Jerry actually took a severed weed and held it back together to see what would happen. The severed halves didn't physically reconnect but the light glowing from the two pieces did. Jerry felt pretty bad chopping weeds after that, but he would do it to keep his stepfather off his back.

There were other times when Jerry had a chance to put his unique abilities on display as a teenager growing up in Kentucky.

One of Jerry's friends, David, had known Jerry for about two years. David knew about Jerry's special abilities and he had tried to copy him a few times, without much success. Jerry was just happy that David didn't think he was weird, and Jerry could just be normal around him.

David also shared Jerry's love of music. On one warm summer day, they were inside an old abandoned home, about to hook up their guitars and play really loud with no one around to complain about it. David's parents owned the then empty house on a plot of land and David had turned it into his clubhouse.

The only problem was that he had established the clubhouse when it was cold. Now it was summertime and wasps had overrun the place.

David warned Jerry that the place was full of wasps, but Jerry said he didn't worry about bugs, "Let's just play music," he said.

"Okay," David said.

But David and Jerry soon realized that their bug problem was serious. Once they started playing music the wasps were everywhere, the wasps' solitude destroyed by the banging of electric guitars. The swarms of wasps buzzing around soon freaked out Jerry and his friend.

34

"Let's get out of here," said David.

"Right behind you," Jerry replied. "But first, I'm going to try something. Hang on a minute, David." Jerry stood in the room a moment, eyes closed, looking like he was concentrating on something. Wasps were landing on him, all over him. Jerry was pulling in all his energy and then he could feel the energy of the wasps. What Jerry did next was something new – he started to absorb all the energy of the wasps – he drained it right out of them. "Okay," Jerry said, "we can leave now."

"What was that all about?" David asked as the left the house.

"You'll see," Jerry replied. "We'll come back in about an hour."

About an hour later, the two boys returned. There wasn't a live wasp anywhere. Instead dozens of dead wasps littered the floor. David was a little freaked out. "What did you do, man?"

"I just took care of your bug problem," Jerry said. "Let's play."

The two hooked up their guitars and began playing. But David was kind of freaked out, and didn't feel like playing for long.

The two remained friends for some time after that, but David had a hard time getting over what Jerry had done. Still, it never caused problems with their friendship. Jerry later told David that it was a wicked thing to do, and he promised to never do it again. Later, David would often tell the wasp story to others, trying to confirm some of the things Jerry could do.

Something else Jerry had a little fun with in those days was remote viewing. It's a well-known phenomenon that came to light during CIA Cold War experiments. The CIA years later admitted it hired psychics who could transport their psychic "vision" in the very deepest recesses of the Kremlin, to find out what the Soviets were up to. As a teenager, Jerry discovered he had the same ability.

Once at school during lunch recess, Jerry closed his eyes, and tried to take a look into a friend's room. "I know what you have hidden under your bed," he told him.

"What?" asked his friend.

"Dirty magazines. If your mom finds out, you're in big trouble," Jerry said.

"How do you know about them? I've never showed you. You've never been in my house. Who told you?" the boy demanded.

"I can see it," Jerry said as he took a bite out of his sandwich. "And that bug you have in a jar on your desk. It's dead. You'd better get rid of it."

The boy's face turned white. "I just caught that thing last night. I didn't tell anyone about it."

"I know," Jerry said. They all had a good laugh at the expense of his friend.

Jerry discovered that if he closed his eyes and focused on a place he could see it in his mind. He was spending a lot of time reading books about places and geography, and that's when he started experimenting with remote viewing. He would close his eyes and think of a place, and then see it in his mind. Then he would look it up in a book to see if he had taken himself to the right place. It was his validation. And it was fun.

Jerry would spend his remaining teenage years in Kentucky, and after graduation he experienced something not uncommon in that part of the world; a shotgun marriage to a girl he had been spending some time with. She wasn't pregnant, not for another year anyway, but Jerry was going to have a family and he needed a job to make some money. He discovered he was good with electronics, so he started fixing things. It was an occupation that would lead him to another remarkable discovery.

Chapter 3
Awakenings

A Healer like Jerry Wills is not someone everyone can accept. Jerry's known that for some time. A lot of people can't open their minds to the possibility that something unable to be dissected by the scientific method could possibly be real. While still others see "healing" as an opportunity for exposing fraud.

There are those out there who firmly believe Jerry Wills and others like him are nothing more than hypnotists tricking people into feeling better for financial gain. Jerry has to be constantly wary of those who will try to trick him. As he freely admits, he can't help everyone. That is especially true when there is nothing really wrong with the person he is treating, or if that person refuses to tell the truth.

After a recent television news report about Jerry, a Phoenix couple called him asking for his services. Both were ill, and doctors weren't helping, they told Jerry. Could they come over right away?

It was only one day after Jerry's story appeared on TV. Jerry and his wife Kathy were taking a lot of calls and scheduling appointments for the following week. But this couple had to see

Jerry right away, so he agreed to see them. They asked Jerry how much he charged.

"I ask for three hundred dollars – if you can't pay that much, that's okay," Jerry said. "Tell you what, since you're a couple, five hundred for both will be fine."

"No problem," was their reply. "Thank you very much. We'll see you tomorrow."

The next day, Jerry drove to their home as planned to see them. They lived in a small but nice home near Sun City on the outskirts of Phoenix. As Jerry pulled in front of the home and parked in the street, he had an uneasy feeling. He sat in his car a few moments, and decided to have a cigarette. He wanted to think about this one, because to him it felt rushed. He didn't like being rushed, didn't like getting into something he wasn't completely sure about. But the couple seemed okay when he talked to them on the phone the day before. So after finishing his cigarette, Jerry got out of the car and walked up to the front door.

After a friendly greeting, the three got down to business. The husband and wife described to Jerry a variety of ailments. She said she believed leaking breast implants were to blame for most of her problems. And her husband blamed arthritis and some other issues with his poor health.

Jerry started with the wife. She sat on a kitchen chair while Jerry moved around to her back. By touching her back, he could see any problems she may have with her chest and leaking implants.

But Jerry discovered something curious. She had no leaking implants. In fact she didn't have any implants at all. Jerry thought it strange, but said only, "I don't see any problems there."

He went on to examine her and her husband. They did have a variety of minor problems; most associated with age. Jerry sent extra energy to those areas in an effort to help the body heal itself.

"I don't see anything major with either of you," he said. "Besides some inflammation, and some pulled muscles here and there, you are both in pretty good health."

They both looked relieved.

"You should feel better in a day or two, so just take it easy and let your bodies heal."

They thanked Jerry, paid him the five hundred dollars, and Jerry left.

Jerry still had a funny feeling about the experience, and he wasn't sure how to feel about the couple he just worked on, because they really had only minor issues with their health.

The next day, Jerry got his answer when the couple called him back.

"We want our money back," the woman demanded. "You are nothing more than a fraud, and we're going to the TV stations to expose you."

Jerry was startled. Putting the pieces together, he thought he might have been victimized by the couple. After all, she lied about her implants. Maybe they were setting him up.

Since they were lying in the first place, Jerry decided not to return their money. "You deceived me about your implants, and everything else that you said was wrong with you," Jerry said. "I will not give you your money back. I did exactly what I was asked to do. Please do not call here again." Jerry hung up the phone.

He worried about the couple for a few days, but never got another phone call, and he was never contacted by the media regarding the couple's allegations of fraud. Because Jerry had been treated so badly by his clients and because he didn't at all like the fact that someone would try to trick him, he started thinking about no longer working as a healer. But the next series of events illustrated to Jerry quite clearly that he had to continue.

A few days after the breast implant incident, Jerry went to see someone in a local Phoenix hospital. An old client turned friend had called for his help. The request was legitimate, much to Jerry's relief, and the healing session went well. The woman was from Flagstaff and had been airlifted to Phoenix with a condition the doctors could not identify. Within fifteen minutes Jerry had solved the mystery. Tests were ordered and proved him correct.

But while he was at the hospital, another couple recognized him from the television story, and asked if he could help their son.

"Sure," Jerry said. "What's the problem?"

"My son had a drug overdose," the woman said. "He hasn't regained consciousness, and doctors are keeping him sedated to avoid brain damage. We're really frightened."

"Okay," Jerry said. "Let me take a look."

A few minutes later he was standing over a teenage boy who was clearly unconscious. Jerry again used a technique he developed over the years to help the boy by improving the energy flow inside his body.

When he was finished, the couple thanked him. "How much should we pay you?" asked the mother as she pulled a checkbook from her purse.

Jerry said, "Oh, don't worry about that. It's on the house."

"Oh, thank you," the woman said again, and kept repeating as she wiped tears from her eyes.

As Jerry was about to leave the hospital room, they all saw the boy began to stir. His parents were shocked to see him waking up.

"Can you hear me?" asked his mother.

"Yes," the boy said, still rather groggy. "Where am I?"

"You're in the hospital," his mother answered. "But you're going to be okay now."

A nurse came into the room, and couldn't understand how the boy was regaining consciousness with all the drugs in his system.

She looked at Jerry. "How did you do that?"

"Oh, it was nothing." Jerry just smiled, and walked from the room.

43

To Jerry, cases like that are what make all the bother and risk worthwhile. To see the look in the faces of the boy's parents was all Jerry needed. It was what keeps him going, keeps him on the path of trying to help people whenever he can.

One time Jerry and his wife Kathy were in Las Vegas for a working vacation. A Las Vegas inspirational TV talk show host, who goes by the name of Matisun, invited Jerry to be on her show and to talk to some people she knew. Her show was called "Matisun TV with Heart."

Matisun, a bubbly, very bright young woman had also written a book, In My Father's Arms, and had produced an inspirational music CD titled "It's a Miracle!"

A friend of Matisun had recommended Jerry for her TV show. Jerry had treated him for a problem with his arm. So Matisun invited both Jerry and Kathy to Las Vegas, offering them free use of her downtown condo if he would be on the show. Jerry agreed and in just a few days was recording a show with Matisun.

There was another reason Matisun had wanted to see Jerry. Twenty years ago Matisun had breast implants, the old kind – silicone. "Intuitively," she told Jerry, "I kind of keep feeling I should have them taken out, but I don't have the courage."

"I'd be happy to take a look," Jerry said.

"I also want my friends to meet you, so you can set up private sessions with them – if that's okay?" she asked Jerry.

"Fine," Jerry said, adding that he looked forward to meeting them.

During her session with Jerry the next afternoon, Matisun told him that she had been wearing a wig.

"My hair is falling out," she said. "I've done some research and I think I have alopecia. I want to do a special show on it, because I discovered thousands of other women have it too."

She also talked to Jerry about the implants.

"Let's check that out first," Jerry said.

As Jerry had done for breast implant exams before, he placed both his hands on Matisun's collarbones and directed his energy down into her breasts.

After only ten seconds, Jerry pulled his hands back. "You have to go right now and call your doctor, and get these things out immediately," he told her. "It has to be done right away."

Even though she suspected a problem with the implants, Matisun looked stunned at the severity of Jerry's warning.

Jerry was also surprised he was so blunt with her. He heard the words coming out of his mouth, but couldn't believe he was saying it. The last thing he wanted to do was scare her but something inside him said he had to warn her, and right away.

"Don't run, but walk, and for God's sake be careful. I want you to walk because if you fall on those things you'll be in big trouble. You have to get those implants out," insisted Jerry. "And you have to do it immediately. Get this done right now." Jerry had rarely been so emphatic about anything, but he knew she was in trouble.

Matisun said she would, and then asked Jerry about her hair. Jerry didn't know what was causing her hair to fall out, but he said he would find out.

"I'm going home and I'm going to pray on what it is," Jerry said. "And I'm going to ask God for a sign of what is making your hair fall out."

Later that night, Jerry and Kathy were up late watching television. Jerry was still thinking about Matisun. Her breast implants worried him and so did her hair loss. While channel surfing the local cable TV offerings, Jerry and Kathy suddenly came across a report on an all-news station that thousands of women were losing their hair because of breast implants.

Jerry immediately picked up the phone and called Matisun.

"That's the connection," he told her after describing what he had seen on TV. "Your hair is falling out because of the implants."

Later, Matisun did her own research and found the proven link between leaky breast implants and alopecia.

A few weeks later, Matisun had the surgery to remove the implants. Her doctor was shocked by what he saw. After the surgery, he told her that her silicone implants could have ruptured at any moment. She could have died if the silicone had spread throughout her body. As he was taking them out, one of the implants just fell apart in his hands. They had to vacuum the silicone breast material, which had spilled into her chest cavity. But the doctor believed they got it all.

Still after all that, there were more complications. Her doctor thought she would have to have more surgery. There was a problem with the skin on her right breast and the doctor told her she might lose part of it.

The first thing Matisun did was call Jerry, who by this time was back home in Phoenix.

"I can work on that over the phone," Jerry said. And he performed another healing session on Matisun right then. Once Jerry had worked on someone in person, it was easy for him to make a reconnection, even over the phone from long distances away.

The next time Matisun saw her doctor, he was amazed. He said he didn't know what Matisun did, but whatever happened, it was a miracle.

"As far as that healing session goes," Matisun later told Jerry, "You saved my life. I'll always be grateful to you because you gave me the impetus to go out and do it."

Matisun continued to suffer hair loss, however. She blamed the heavy metals and other toxins still in her system as a result of the implants, and possibly from the implant that ruptured during surgery. Until it clears up, she's decided to shave her head. But she gives most of the credit to Jerry for saving her life, telling friends that it was the best decision she ever made.

"You know what I love about Jerry?" she said. "It's his genuine longing and passion to be in service that way. To help others make their own connections. He genuinely cares and he genuinely wants to be of service. He genuinely connects to that place where miracles happen. I definitely felt I was in the presence of a great spirit."

The decision to become a healer in the first place wasn't an easy one for Jerry. It was a process that began years before, shortly after his shotgun marriage ended, and he was married a second time.

He decided that life on the farm wasn't what he wanted, so Jerry went into electronics. Jerry seemed to be a natural when it came to fixing electronic gadgets and appliances and eventually opened his own business which at first was very successful.

Now he was happily married, with children, and a successful businessman. What could be better? He knew his psychic abilities and healing powers were still a part of him, but he considered psychic phenomena a realm already occupied, leaving little room for him.

Besides, he really didn't need it. His new wife and family weren't fond of the subject in the first place, so Jerry went on a mission to fulfill his vision of the great American dream – a vision even Jerry admits was self-serving: A good career, money to spend, a home and a family. Why couldn't he be like everyone else?

He became very self-serving and quite focused on being successful. He didn't want to be a mean person, but he wanted to be a shrewd business person. His goal was to succeed at all costs, whatever it took.

Jerry got the idea, of all places, by watching the CBS TV prime time soap opera, "Dallas". At the time, Jerry was young and impressionable and doing everything he could do to get ahead. On "Dallas", the main character, JR, seemed to get whatever he needed and went forward, always forward…and that's what Jerry wanted. Even though JR's drive ultimately led to his own demise, Jerry didn't look at it that way.

But then the economy of rural Michigan took a spiral downwards, and Jerry's second wife left him.

He decided to pack up and move to Phoenix, Arizona. Why, he wasn't sure. But like so many others who moved west at the time, it seemed like a good place for a fresh start on life.

Like many young men who pulled up stakes, Jerry struggled just to make ends meet. He was in a strange city, and he had no friends. He was working as an electronics repairman for a large department store. Workers were expected to repair at least eight televisions or stereos a week. Jerry was fixing ten or twelve a day. They didn't like that, because Jerry was making everyone else look bad. So they fired him.

Jerry worked odd jobs after that, most in electronics repair. But he did meet a man who would become his best friend.

As they got to know each other, Jerry learned that Neil Miller was acquainted with the burgeoning 1980's New Age community of Phoenix, Arizona. Neil and his roommate John also studied hypnosis and were fascinated with the people conducting channeling sessions in the Phoenix area.

Simply put, channeling is the New Age concept for mediums in which a spirit speaks through a medium of their choosing.

After learning about Jerry's special abilities like remote viewing and seeing energy, Neil suggested Jerry try channeling. Both were fascinated by all New Age concepts, but Jerry held back. He wasn't convinced that channeling would be good for him. However, they did agree to go see a man who was channeling an entity named Dr. Peebles. The medium's name was Kevin Ryerson, who would later became world famous and appear as himself in the film Out on a Limb starring Shirley MacLaine. Ryerson had four spirit guides, including the 17th century Irish doctor called Dr.

Peebles. The other three were a Nubian slave, a witchdoctor from Haiti and the Biblical John.

But long before gaining any real fame, Ryerson was holding sessions in a small Phoenix venue amazing people with his connection with Dr. Peebles.

One night, Jerry and Neil attended one of Ryerson's sessions. Jerry thought Ryerson looked like a Fancy Dan, and watched as Ryerson sat there with his eyes rolled back in his head and talking in a brogue Irish accent.

"This is fascinating," Jerry told Neal.

They both listened intently as Ryerson told his audience what was wrong with them and what they could do to help themselves.

Jerry and Neil stayed in the back of the room just watching Ryerson. They tried to talk to him afterwards, but after fighting through a crowd of people, Ryerson stopped talking as soon as he saw Jerry and just walked away. Jerry thought it was odd but didn't think about it too much.

They went back a second time, and again they were both amazed by Ryerson's channeling session with Dr. Peebles. This time Ryerson was seeing people around him, people that Jerry was seeing, too. Jerry had been able to see "dead people" since he was a child, but he thought it was natural, believing that everyone could. Later he learned to ignore them. After all, they didn't bother Jerry all that much. Not yet, anyway.

After watching yet another Ryerson channeling session, Jerry tried again to talk to him. He came up to Ryerson and asked, "How do you do that?"

But Ryerson wouldn't answer. He just looked at Jerry and said nothing – just like the other time.

"Why do you do that? Why do you clam up?" Jerry asked.

"Because you can do this; you don't need me," Ryerson said, in a very dismissive tone. "These people can't do it. They need me."

"If I can do it," Jerry asked, "how do I do it?"

Ryerson looked away and said, "When the student is ready, the teacher will appear."

"Who taught you?" Jerry asked.

"Doctor Richard Ireland." It was all Ryerson had to say.

That was about all Jerry got out of him. It was a disappointing encounter, but it only encouraged Jerry to dig deeper into the mystery.

Neil Miller, as curious about channeling as Jerry, wanted to see if his friend with obvious psychic and healing gifts could channel anyone. So he continued to ask Jerry if he could hypnotize him. Jerry remained uncertain. He still felt uncomfortable. But one night Jerry said okay. After he got drowsy, they could try a channeling session.

Pamela, Jerry's girlfriend at the time, was studying to become a court reporter. They decided to have her attend so she could take notes of whatever Jerry came up with. Neither of them had any kind of voice recorder.

Soon Jerry was sleepy, and Neil decided the time was right to put him into hypnosis.

Two hours later, Jerry woke up. His girlfriend had pages and pages of material from a person who Jerry had channeled while he was in hypnosis.

While he was under, Neil had asked the entity to identify itself. The entity Jerry was channeling said he could be called M.

"M, like in Michael?" asked Neil.

"Yes, like Michael," replied M.

For two hours the entity had discussed his past lives, the supernatural, and energy healing. Neil Miller and Jerry's girlfriend were fascinated by the conversation.

Jerry was surprised to hear all this after he woke up. He had no recollection of it, and the experience left him less interested in channeling. After all, he hadn't gotten anything out of it, besides a good nap.

It continued to be a tough personal time for Jerry. He drifted in and out of jobs. At one point he lost his apartment and moved in with Neil. His dreams of a successful family and professional life seemed to vanish in front of him. But Neil was always supportive. He was always positive and always had something good to say. He tried to help Jerry any way he could.

Jerry was looking for answers; so was Neil. But Jerry wanted to look beyond channeling because he wasn't getting anything out of it. They both decided to go see Ryerson's teacher, Dr. Richard Ireland.

Ireland first became aware of his psychic abilities at the age of five, following eye surgery. When a nurse found him bouncing a ball off the wall of his hospital room, she rushed in to find out why he had removed the bandages covering both eyes. She was amazed to discover he hadn't. It was the beginning of Dr. Richard Ireland's awareness...what he called his "x-ray clairvoyance, a certain sensory sight without physical vision."

Ireland's professional career as a psychic began when he started to demonstrate his abilities to scholars and scientists at the University of Southern Oregon, the University of Arizona and Arizona State University in Tempe. Dr. Ireland was even invited to act as a consultant in the selection and training for NASA's manned space program. Ireland also established what others called the first known "New Age" church in America.

In 1980, Dr. Richard Ireland was holding psychic performances at a hotel which is now the Red Roof Inn on Camelback Road in West Phoenix. One Saturday night, Neil invited Jerry to go with him and offered to pay, knowing Jerry had little extra income at the time. Jerry, remembering that

Kevin Ryerson had told him Dr. Ireland was his teacher, decided to go.

Ireland had a lounge act at the Inn, and at first Jerry thought the whole thing must be a scam.

Jerry and Neil stood there looking at an overweight man in a white shirt with a black jacket and black jeans. Ireland also looked old and tired, with thinning hair and an ashen complexion.

As Jerry watched, Ireland put cotton balls over his eyes and taped them in place. Jerry was thinking he's sure this guy has an angle; there's got to be something going on. He's a magician or something. He's got everyone buffaloed.

But as Jerry and Neil watched, Ireland walked through the darkened nightclub with about eighty-five people seated around him. Everyone was silent because Ireland's got their attention. He was still blindfolded, walking around through rows of tables and chairs, walking up to people in the audience as if he could see them, but he didn't bump into anyone or anything. As Jerry now watched in awe, Ireland even stepped over a lady's bag, and then leaned over to Neil to say something.

Ireland revealed Neil's girlfriend's phone number, the type of car she drove, and her driver's license number. Everything Ireland said was correct, right on the money. Neil and Jerry were amazed. Ireland was accurate about everything he said as he moved from person to person.

Stunned, not knowing what to think, Jerry continued to watch as Ireland asked for a volunteer. Intrigued, Jerry was the first to raise his hand.

"There's a fellow right there," Ireland, still wearing his blindfold, pointed directly to Jerry. "Come on up here." Ireland was facing the other direction, but pointed right at Jerry.

Jerry stood and made his way to the front of the room. He walked up on stage left. Ireland was standing stage right.

"Do you want me to read the numbers off that five dollar bill in your pocket?" Ireland asked.

Jerry thought, hah, I have him now! "I don't have a five dollar bill," Jerry said. He knew he had a one-dollar bill he was saving for a Coke, but there was no five dollar bill in his wallet.

"If I can read the numbers off that five dollar bill, can I have it?" Ireland asked.

"If I have a five dollar bill," Jerry replied.

"You do."

"No, I don't," Jerry said, as the audience chuckled, getting amused by the scene on stage.

Jerry pulled his pockets out, and showed Ireland the one-dollar bill he was saving.

"I don't want that," Ireland said. "I know you have a dollar. I'm not going to take that. That's going to be for when you leave here. You are going to buy a drink."

Jerry thought, whoa...how does he know that?

"Pull out your wallet," Ireland commanded. "It's in your right back pocket."

"Okay," Jerry said as he reached behind him and pulled out his billfold from his right back pocket. Jerry showed the crowd it had some papers and his license, but no five-dollar bill.

"My God," Ireland said, "do I have to take you through every step to find this five-dollar bill? Too bad it's not a twenty."

The audience laughed out loud.

"I don't have a five dollar bill," insisted Jerry.

"Yes, you do. Start digging through that thing."

Jerry began to take papers out of his wallet, and to his amazement, there it was: a five-dollar bill folded and tucked behind some old receipts. He thought, oh shit, I have five bucks. I could have had something to drink already.

The audience applauded as Jerry held up the five.

"Okay," Ireland said, "If I read the numbers off that five dollar bill, it's mine."

He thought, oh, I'm screwed. "Fine," Jerry said.

"Do you want me to read it backwards or forwards?" Ireland asked.

"Backwards," Jerry said.

Ireland read the numbers, correctly, backwards. "Do you want me to read it forwards now?"

"Sure."

Ireland read the five-dollar bill's serial numbers...forward.

As Jerry nodded to the applauding crowd, Ireland walked over and without missing a beat, snatched the five out of Jerry's fingers. He then crumpled it, and dropped it on the floor. "I've got so many of these. You're dismissed!"

Jerry walked off the stage, his head spinning. He made it a point right then to go see this guy. He had to know more.

Doctor Richard Ireland passed away before explaining to Jerry exactly how he worked his special psychic abilities, what he called his "x-ray clairvoyance." But Jerry did get one opportunity to meet him off stage.

Ireland once commented to Jerry at another one of his shows that they should get together and talk, so Jerry invited himself to a gathering of Dr. Ireland's friends in Scottsdale one weekend afternoon. It was an afternoon cup of coffee kind of party, something Jerry felt comfortable attending.

Jerry and the others arrived first. He felt mostly out of place. The large well-furnished Scottsdale home was full of men in suits and women in nice dresses. Jerry felt out of place in his jeans and t-shirt.

When dogs started barking in the yard, Jerry took a look out the window. The Doctor was arriving, in a chauffeured driven white limousine, the kind common in Las Vegas at the time.

As Jerry watched, the driver got out and walked around to the rear passenger door and opened it, and out came Dr. Richard Ireland.

The aging, overweight psychic rose slowly out of the back seat and straightened up. Ireland took a moment to adjust his vest, and make sure his shirt was tucked in. He had on one of those vests that ended in a point on either side. Ireland also wore a large white hat that was kind of cocked off to one side. Sunglasses completed the look.

Ireland walked slowly up to the house, and everyone was happy to see him. Jerry hung back for awhile, not wanting to force the issue.

But soon Ireland walked over to Jerry and remembered his name.

"Hello again, Jerry," he said.

"Hello, Doctor. Thanks for inviting me…sort of."

Ireland chuckled. "I'm glad you could make it." He pulled Jerry aside and they ended up outside on a backyard patio. They sat and talked for a while.

Jerry discovered that Ireland was a very easy person to talk to. But he didn't go into a lot of details about his private life, nor did he explain to Jerry how he did what he does.

"I can tell you I'm not allowed to go to Las Vegas," Ireland said. "They won't let me play there. But do you want me to give you some lottery numbers?" he asked Jerry.

Jerry laughed. "No, that's okay," Jerry said. It was a response he would later regret.

"Suit yourself," Ireland said.

Jerry said he wanted to do what Dr. Ireland did. Jerry thought it would be great.

But Ireland shook his head no. "I've known all along that I'm here for entertainment. You, on the other hand, are here for another reason. You are here to help people. That's far beyond entertainment."

After a few minutes, Ireland got up and said, "They are probably wondering where I've gone off to. I've got to go."

Jerry decided he might as well leave, too. There was no reason for him to stay.

Jerry saw Ireland again a couple of years later during a similar nightclub performance. He saw his limousine around town a few times, but the two never got the chance to speak like that again.

His talk with Ireland helped Jerry in other ways, however; it validated that he was having similar experiences. Up to that point, everything Jerry had done was purely subjective. He had no way to gauge what he was experiencing, what he had experienced as a child and what he was experiencing now as a young adult, twenty-eight years old. Ireland was someone who absolutely blew Jerry's mind with what he could do. The stories about Ireland had gone far beyond what Jerry had seen, so the validation was significant. It was letting him know that, yes, there was something to all this.

Ireland gave Jerry a reason to look deeper because up to that point in time, being involved in anything that was metaphysical or unseen was at best a shade of gray away from sleight of hand. He couldn't really put his finger on whether what he was encountering was actually real, or just a good trick. Richard Ireland gave him a reason to keep looking, just by virtue of the fact that to Jerry he was so matter of fact about it, and he was so down to Earth.

About a year later Jerry landed a job as an electronics systems designer and was assigned to install a new sound system at a graduate campus in Glendale, Arizona, called Thunderbird, the Garvin School of International Management. The school was founded in 1946 on the site of an old World War II pilot training facility. The runways, hangars and control tower made up the original campus, and much of it still stands today. In 1981, some of its hangars were still being converted into classrooms when Jerry got the job.

Jerry didn't like his employers much, but at least the job gave Jerry some cash in his pocket, and he was able to move back into his own place.

Jerry was assigned to build a sound system that would allow every classroom on campus to be able to hear the same public-address announcements. The module he constructed was filled with electronic components inside a chest that weighed more than six hundred pounds.

After testing it and pronouncing it ready, workers had hauled the chest and installed it in the upper reaches of one of the aircraft hangars - a good fifty feet above the hangar floor. The large, multi-component filled box was held in place by a small wooden platform built just to hold it.

But right away, the unit malfunctioned. It was November 11th, 1981, at eleven o'clock in the morning, and Jerry was back on the job site. Others who had tried to operate the sound system said it didn't work right. So Jerry had to figure out what was going wrong.

Jerry's boss had already placed a ladder to the platform. And it was the longest ladder Jerry had ever seen, reaching all the way to the platform more than fifty feet high.

Jerry noticed that one of the feet at the end of the ladder was missing, and he mentioned it to his supervisor. His response was, "Get the hell up there and fix the God damned thing if you want to keep your job."

Jerry needed the work, and the money, so reluctantly he headed up the shaky ladder. Carefully climbing to keep his balance, and to keep the ladder from tipping over, Jerry eventually made it back to the top of the hangar to check his custom made sound system.

His right foot eventually found a secure place on the platform, and he slowly removed the bolts securing the front panel and gave it a slight tug. The panel slid forward a few inches but stopped. Something was still connected at the rear. In his rush to finish the job and get back down the ladder, Jerry had forgotten to disconnect the cables behind the front panel first. His hands trembled as he reached behind the cabinet and removed the first wiring harness. The second was further from his reach, so at an uncomfortable angle, Jerry reached further behind the chest to free the last harness.

But his left foot slid away from him, and the ladder began moving, twisting back and forth while Jerry tried to hold his balance. Before he could react, the entire platform started to tilt and give way. Hanging almost in midair between the ladder and the platform itself, Jerry had nowhere to go but down. His blood ran cold as he reached for the corner of the steel chest in desperation. It was pointless. The ladder began to fall, and the platform with it. Jerry was falling, too, and in that instant he remembered looking down, hoping the distance wasn't so great, and that perhaps there would be a safe place to land. He only felt the sensation of free fall before blacking out. His scream and parts of the platform were all that hung in the air.

What happened next can only be described as a near-death experience, one that would affect Jerry for the rest of his life.

After entering what seemed to be a timeless darkness at the start of his fall, Jerry instantly became aware of a light, some movement and the sound of voices. The voices seemed to surround him, and the more Jerry focused, the less he was concerned with falling or the life threatening consequences he faced.

Instantly he became aware that the conversation he was hearing, and now seeing, was between himself and another person. Jerry remembered the exchange; it was something from his past. Jerry had lied and manipulated the person he was talking to so the man would feel sorry for him. "The alarming difference was," Jerry said, "that within the exchange, this time I was on the receiving end of my actions. I felt the sense of betrayal and emotional pain I caused. It felt so awful to know I had done this to someone who trusted me."

In another such vision, Jerry saw himself back in Kentucky on his way to church. He was just a child and was attending Sunday service with the neighbor's kids. As he entered the church, Jerry held the door open for an old lady. He held it open for her; she came in and thanked the tall, young man before her. Jerry then let the door close and took his seat.

As Jerry recalled, "The reason I opened the door for her was because I wanted to gain good favor with God, not because I wanted to help her. I thought this will give me some points, which is a typical juvenile thing. Still, it must have registered out there somewhere."

Each time Jerry watched an exchange or event from his past (his life was literally passing before his eyes) it quickly faded and was immediately replaced by another one. And in every case, Jerry was at the receiving end of his actions. He was ashamed and felt deep regret over what he had said or done. "The times I had done a nice thing for someone were only because I thought it would further my cause," he said. "The times I had acted charitably were only because I want to be recognized as a charitable person. Each occasion played itself out fully, allowing me to experience what an awful person I had been. My heart was broken time and time again, by me."

There were only one or two truly positive memories played out before Jerry's eyes. One was during his first wife's birthday. They had no money, and Jerry pawned his high school ring to get her a present. To him, it was no big deal. But when he experienced it through his wife's perspective, he regained a sense of how important it was to her.

He also experienced joy through the perspective of his children. "When you have kids you don't put yourself in their place and think how good it feels to be held by someone…but now I had a sense of how it felt from my daughter when I was holding her and just laughing and singing to her when I was being playful with her. I got to sense that, and it was wonderful."

But the negative feelings Jerry had just experienced left him deeply troubled and saddened.

"I desperately wanted to go to each person and ask forgiveness. I desperately wanted to hold each of those who loved me. I wanted to tell them how much they meant to me," Jerry said. "Somewhere deep inside whatever I was now, I knew it was over. My chance was gone. I was, after a twenty-eight year lifetime, left with only regret. I vowed to myself I would never allow such regret again. I supposed it would be remembered at some point in my next incarnation because I knew I was going to die."

In the very next instant, Jerry became aware of himself all over again. He was now floating above the scene on the hangar floor. Below him was his body lying flat on the ground, a few boards and rubbish scattered around him and near his remains. "I felt detached as I observed the events unfolding beneath me," he said.

Several people ran towards the body, and Jerry heard their screams as each one yelled, "Call 911! Call 911!"

But Jerry felt a sense of peace and comfort beyond anything he knew in his lifetime. "It seems strange now to think about the detachment I felt," Jerry explained later. "It was wonderful, peaceful and comfortable. I realized how much more I could have accomplished with so little effort, had I tried. Yet, I was at peace with this as I watched the men touch my body, searching for a pulse. In the distance I heard sirens, and I guessed they were for me."

But his time in a pleasant, pain-free existence would be short lived. Soon, Jerry became aware of another presence. Though he could not see anyone else, he knew he was not alone.

Then a voice came through clear and distinctly, "Jerry, what are you doing here?"

Jerry felt soothed hearing the voice, but for some reason he never looked around to see who was talking. He just kept looking at the scene beneath him. Jerry answered, "I fell. And I guess I'm dead now."

"Jerry, you aren't supposed to be here yet."

"Well, I'm here." Jerry said. "I'm not really sure what I'm supposed to do."

"You have to go back, Jerry. You aren't supposed to be here yet. You have something to do. You have to go back, Jerry."

"No," Jerry replied. "I feel pretty good right here. I don't think I want to go back. Look at that. I'm down there dead! I feel pretty good right now. I think I'll stay."

"No. You can't stay, Jerry," insisted the voice once more. "You have to go back…right now!"

It was as if Jerry had been blasted from a cannon. The force was incredible. Panic raced through his body as he lurched and gasped for air. Slowly air filled his lungs, but all he felt was pain.

"I was gasping, gasping, trying to breathe. I couldn't breathe. I was starting to flop and jerk on the floor," Jerry said.

People came running up to him, mostly other construction workers also in the hangar. Most of them told Jerry to lie still, to stop moving.

Jerry was thinking, "Oh, my God, what is going on? What happened?" He began to drift in and out of consciousness. He was soon in the back of an ambulance, on his way to the closest hospital. Jerry woke up once or twice, and remembers wearing a neck brace. He also remembers his arrival at the hospital and the quick trip to the x-ray machine. "Finally I came to my senses, thinking about what had just happened. I remembered how it was before I'd left the farm, and sort of reflecting on what had happened to me morally and emotionally afterwards. Then I made a resolution that I would never do anything again that would put me in a position where I would be on the other end of my actions, and experience anything that I did that was bad, hurtful, rude or otherwise deceitful or inappropriate."

The "J. R. Ewing" inside Jerry was gone. The desire to get ahead, no matter what the cost, had vanished. And he couldn't help but immediately think back on the past experiences he had just relived. "It was so vivid. Every sequence was vivid, like waking up from an extremely lucid dream. It remains now, even years later, very vivid."

There was another side effect of Jerry's fall. Whether psychological or due to brain trauma, Jerry couldn't remember anything from the last ten years.

"I couldn't remember what my ex-wife looked like. I couldn't remember friends. I could barely remember events that were obviously associated with me because I saw the pictures," Jerry said. "It was as if that part was taken away from me so completely that it's as if it had happened to someone else."

Jerry rationalized that he had gone through a death sequence and that part of his life that was the worst part was just deleted. "You don't need to think about this. It was kind of like a past life thing. People don't remember their past lives, why? Well, what good is it going to do you anyway?"

Jerry did not miss most things about his past. It was as if he were brand new again – re-born. He did remember many of the good things, but it was sketchy. "I don't have a color picture to put it with," he explained. "The doctors said maybe I had some brain damage. They said the brain isn't designed to take that kind of impact and survive. They said I was very lucky to be alive."

Lucky, yes. Broken up, certainly. Jerry's x-rays showed he had a variety of broken bones, a concussion and one very big hole in his hand. "When I fell, I must have grabbed something and it put a hole in my hand, a big hole. They had it all bandaged up and it was seeping blood. They had tubes in it to drain it." The doctors told Jerry he would be in the hospital for a while. They didn't say when he might be able to leave.

But Jerry's misery didn't last long. He woke up the next day feeling tired of the whole thing, and surprisingly he felt pretty good. When a nurse came in to change the bandage on his hand, it had miraculously healed. There was no hole, only a raw red spot where the hole used to be. There was no bleeding, no need to drain anything.

"My, don't we heal fast?" the amazed nurse said.

Later, Jerry got out of bed. He stood for a moment, still not feeling any pain. He began to stretch, turning this way and that. "A sensor on my neck was annoying me, so I took it off and started popping my neck," Jerry said. "I was twisting and turning, and reaching over my head. And then the doctor walked in."

At first, the doctor flipped out, and told Jerry he couldn't do that. And he started to list all the things that Jerry had broken. "You have a broken neck," he said. "You're going to be a paraplegic if you keep doing that. Lie down right now!" The doctor then called a nurse to take Jerry to the x-ray department immediately.

"They took me into x-ray again, and x-rayed me there," Jerry says. After examining his second round of x-rays, his doctor could find nothing wrong.

Amazed, the doctor had no explanation. To Jerry, it was just something that happened, nothing more. He thinks it was just part of God's plan. "The whole thing was to put me back on track again," he says. "There was no reason for me to be broken up for any length of time."

But even after the second set of x-rays, his doctor still wanted Jerry to stay hospitalized, at least until he could figure out what was going on.

Jerry didn't think that was a good idea. However, he had no clothes, so he called Neil and Pam and asked them to bring him some new clothes and a pack of cigarettes and a lighter. They had cut off his clothes and had thrown his cigarettes away when he arrived the day before.

Jerry told the doctors he was going home, and as soon as his friend showed up, he did just that. But only after doctors gave him a bag of drugs to treat the pain they were sure he must be in.

Soon Jerry was dressed, outside, having a cigarette and holding a bag of drugs. "It was literally a large brown paper bag filled with stuff. They said I had to take the bag with me, so I did. I signed myself out, went to the nearest dumpster, and threw it in there. I lit up a cigarette and went home."

Jerry felt a bit stiff and a little sore in a few places. But other than that, he was fine.

When Jerry got home, there was a letter waiting for him from his second wife – requesting he give up guardianship of their child Jonathan to her new husband. "What a thing to come home to," Jerry said, "after nearly dying."

The whole experience taught him one very important lesson. "We have to be aware of how our actions impact others," Jerry learned. "That an act of kindness is never wasted, and doing something good, even though it doesn't seem like it at the time, makes a difference. It doesn't mean there is more good in the world; it just means there is less bad."

Experiencing what it felt like on the other side of his life was the key. "Being on the other end of a kindness that you've offered is very gratifying. We all like to think we are good people, but when you are on the other end of the situation, when you are the victim of a real jerk, that's a real eye opener, especially when you feel their pain. When you feel that hurt, there is no hurt that you've ever experienced that matches the hurt of another person from some action that you've taken, especially when it was done deceitfully. So yes, I learned a huge lesson from that. I don't want to go to the other side and have to relive that one again. That would be just awful."

But when you've done something nice for someone? Jerry says it gives that person a sense of value. And a sense of value can change a person's life completely. It can give them a reason to take the next step, or maybe a few more steps and do something great. "What it does for you," Jerry said, "is give you a sense that you are okay, but what it does for them – it can really change their lives in very unpredictable ways."

Jerry believes the experience equals what many people refer to as karma. "When you go through something like that, you have to find it within yourself to forgive yourself. And that's hard to do."

Besides that, Jerry said, "Of all the lessons I have learned, I can tell you with certainty that love is the greatest experience you will ever know."

The near-death experience did more than give Jerry a new appreciation for the way he treated others. It also did more than erase the bad memories of the past ten years or so. The experience left him with a guide. Not the person who told him that it wasn't his time to go. It was someone else, the same person his friend Neil had brought to the surface during Jerry's first channeling session. He was M...no longer an entity that only surfaced during hypnosis. M was now talking to Jerry while he dreamed, and while he was awake.

Jerry's first waking encounter with M came just one night after his fall. "I thought I was dreaming," Jerry said. "I was having a conversation with this person. And the dreams continued on for a number of months, on and off. It was always the same person I was talking to and it was always the same kind of tone and tempo to the conversation. It was like I was having a dream with another person, but I wasn't dreaming." Clearly it was unusual, even for a person like Jerry, to have repeated dreams with the same person. And each dream and every conversation was different.

Sometimes M showed up in the middle of the night, once when Jerry and his wife Kathy were up late talking.

Jerry remembers having a normal conversation with his wife, when suddenly, Jerry heard Kathy say, "No, don't stop now."

Jerry said, "Stop what? What are you talking about?"

"I was having a conversation with M," Kathy said.

It was 2:30 in the morning. Jerry had no idea it had gotten so late. Apparently, he had fallen off to sleep, but M kept talking.

"I tried to keep it from happening," Jerry said. "Because I don't find it to be something I can put credibility to. And if I'm not there having a good time with it myself, what's the point? I'm just channeling like all these other people are channeling, and I don't think that's what I'm here for."

The search for answers led Jerry to many other people, some of whom became his greatest guides for truth and knowledge. In Jerry's words, they took him deeper down the rabbit hole.

But it was M who put Jerry on the path toward becoming a healer.

There is no more important voyage for Jerry than the one M took him on one evening shortly after his near death experience.

M doesn't just talk to Jerry. Sometimes he takes him to strange and wonderful places. Once, he took Jerry to a beautiful countryside setting, with big blocks of stone arranged like an amphitheater. Dozens of other people were there, too, of all races. "There must have been fifty to sixty others sitting around this pavilion-like setting," Jerry explained. "Everyone was just sitting there with their own version of M. Then the strangest thing happened. This guy just appears on a flattened stone and he starts this lecture. He talks about how to be the best that you can be. He talked about protecting our existence by being the most loving and gracious that you can be. I've integrated a lot of this stuff that I heard that night into the talks that I give."

For Jerry, it's hard to put into words exactly what was said. "It was like a dream," he said, "but it was so real."

The experience continued – and as Jerry said, grew even stranger. "We're still sitting there, and a few seconds later, this fellow is gone. He just fades out like a point of light. I look around and all these other people are gone too."

Jerry turned and said to M, "Aren't we going, too?"

M said, "Not yet. There's someone who wants to talk to you."

Suddenly there was a bright light. Jerry had trouble looking at it. "This magnesium-like fire is just sitting there in front of me. Suddenly, it's a person. I'm looking at him, and he turns to look at me, but I could not look at his eyes. It was so bright that it's almost like the sun reflecting off a car bumper. It wasn't painful, but it was so intense there was no way I could look at this person."

Jerry said to M, "Who is that?"

"That's the Father."

"That's God?" Jerry asked.

"That's God," M replied.

"Why would God want to talk to me?"

"That's the Father," M repeated.

"I don't get it."

"Look," said M, "it's like that's the Father and you're the son."

Jerry said, "Okay, but what about everyone else? Aren't they his children?"

"Exactly," said M. "Now you've got it. You've had a chance to witness the Father. They haven't. So let them know He's real."

Jerry then turned to the presence who had joined them and said, "If you're God, I have some questions for you."

M laughed. "I told you so!"

The person M had identified as God then said to Jerry, "What would you like to know?"

Jerry then asked what most people would ask under similar circumstances. After all, he was standing face to face with the Almighty. "What's the meaning of life?"

M laughed again.

The Father said, "There isn't a meaning to life. That's the whole meaning of it."

"I don't get it."

"As soon as you put a meaning to it you've defeated the purpose of it."

"So just going from one experience to another experience to another experience…that's the purpose of life?" asked Jerry.

"No, that's part of the process." The Father then went on to tell Jerry that, "You have life, so you have a chance to grow through your experiences and understand how valuable some things are to embrace, and how valuable some things are to release."

"Like loving each other and caring about each other and so forth?"

"Yes, exactly. The things you understand, those decisions that you make about the things you want to avoid that you don't want to be a part of your life…you can go and have those experiences so you'll understand why you don't want them. It's all a process of your growth. You are there to be there in my place."

"Why don't you do it? Why aren't you there?" asked Jerry.

"I'm there looking at you when you meet someone, and I'm there looking at them when they meet you. You have to understand that you are all part of what I am and I'm part of what you are. We are all connected and growing together."

The conversation between the entity M described as "The Father" and Jerry went on for some time. As Jerry recalled, "A lot of the things I was hearing from him I had no exposure to at the time. But later, as I learned more, I was hearing the same message over and over again from other people. It was really interesting because now I had a point of reference, knowing that these people had truly made the same connection to the Creator."

Whether Jerry Wills had a real face to face with God is something neither he nor anyone else can ever prove. The most important point of the conversation is that Jerry believes it happened, and what Jerry took from the experience forever changed his life. "I learned the Creator wasn't out there somewhere. The Creator was always inside. M said, 'Where do you think you are?' I said, 'I'm not sure where I am. Maybe this is heaven. Or maybe this is what it looks like when you are outside looking in.'"

Chapter Four
Discoveries

Although not widely known as a healer, Jerry continued to explore his special abilities after his nearly fatal fifty-foot fall from the top of an airplane hangar. Jerry and his best friend Neil Miller continued to attend meetings and gatherings where anything paranormal was the norm. To make a living, Jerry continued to repair electronic devices, but he knew there had to be something more.

Then Jerry made another friend, his name was Randy Winters. He had once traveled to Switzerland to interview and personally investigate the UFO sighting claims made by Billy Meier. At that time, Randy was considered an authority on what would become known as the Meier alien contacts.

Meier was a world famous UFO witness who claimed personal contact, and had taken authenticated photos of extraterrestrial craft operated by a race of aliens known as the Pleiadians.

Randy Winters had been investigating UFO sightings since 1979. He had done the first serious work on the Meier's sightings and is author of a book <u>The Pleiadian Mission</u>.

Randy and Jerry became good friends, and Jerry was invited to speak at a gathering of paranormal investigators in Wisconsin. Another paranormal investigator, Virgil Armstrong, was invited to speak there, too.

As a result of Jerry's appearance at these and other events, he became a favorite of the paranormal speaking circuit. The highlight was an all expense paid trip to Berlin, as the guest of co-speaker Virgil Armstrong.

For Jerry, the trip to Germany was a wild, noisy event. If the Germans didn't agree with you, they stood up and shouted, "No, I don't think so."

They'll tell you their view and challenge you. But when Jerry was up there to speak, a huge hall filled with hundreds of people was eerily silent. It was very different than what other speakers experienced. Nobody said a word as Jerry talked about his experiences.

People were sitting on the floor; others were standing. The hall was filled to capacity. There were even people outside the building listening on a loud speaker system.

Jerry learned during his experience in Germany and speaking at other venues that for some reason when he speaks, people listen. It may go back to his demeanor. Most people find his slow, calm, thoughtful delivery almost spellbinding.

Jerry doesn't consider the message he delivers that ground breaking. It is nothing more than that you are more than the sum of your parts.

He doesn't recognize it for being a big deal, just common sense.

Time and time again at various conferences, people would come up to Jerry afterwards and say he was the most perfect speaker that they had listened to in a long time. They would ask Jerry if he was a member of Toastmasters. And ask how did he learn to control a crowd like that?

Jerry tells them, "I just say what I have to say."

Jerry says part of the credit goes to his lack of pretense. "If you like me, you like me," he told a member of his audience one time. "If you don't, you don't. I'm just me, and I can be comfortable about being me without being worried about whether someone likes me or not. I think a lot of people are concerned about how well they are received. So they try to be what they expect the other folks would appreciate, and I don't. If they don't like me, then that's good, too."

One of the most important speaking engagements Jerry ever accepted was in Austin, Texas. He was about thirty-five years old at the time. Jerry was invited to present a lecture to the Austin paranormal group. There were several doctors and nurses in attendance. It was set up at an Austin Holiday Inn, a very nice place. And Jerry enjoyed his visit and the reaction he got from several medical professionals. He actually worked on a couple of people in front of them, and they were amazed at the positive results they all had. To

Jerry it was a very satisfying trip, because it again provided some validation for what he was doing.

Whether Jerry's demonstrations had any impact on future healers in the area is impossible to tell. But according to the website, www.austinholistic.com, there are currently twenty-seven "Energy Healers" listed in the Austin area.

Later the hosts of the event invited Jerry to their home. They had a log cabin guesthouse for Jerry to stay in overlooking a river that ran through town. It had a nice view, and Jerry accepted happily.

Little did Jerry know, but his hosts had invited a special guest to see him. Later that evening while Jerry was relaxing with his hosts just before sunset, a tall woman with short white hair came walking up to him. She wore an ankle-length white dress, and had to be about fifty-five years old. She had a special presence about her though, thought Jerry. A man who Jerry learned later was her doctor had come along as well.

The woman walked up to Jerry and said, "I have uterine cancer, and you have to help me."

"Okay," Jerry said, "Give me a minute, and we'll get after it."

Her doctor told Jerry that the prognosis wasn't good. His patient was refusing any kind of surgery or chemotherapy and if left untreated she would die, period. He also told Jerry it would be a miserable death.

82

The woman agreed. "It will be a miserable death," she said, "because I'm not doing that shit."

They continued to talk as Jerry finished his cigarette; smoking helped Jerry calm himself and prepare for a healing session.

"What do you do here?" Jerry asked her.

"I'm a healer," she said. "I have been since I was a little girl. But I can't heal myself." It's a problem common with most healers, she explains. She can't become an observer of her own problem. "My friends say you are a gifted healer," she said to Jerry. "I hope you can help me."

"I'll do what I can," Jerry said. He stood next to her and held his hands a few inches from her stomach.

"What are you doing?" she asked.

Up until that point, Jerry had not placed his hands on anyone he was healing. He put his hands near people but just a couple of inches off their clothes. He never touched them. As described earlier in this book, Jerry's unwillingness to touch someone was most likely an inherent reaction to being scolded as a child. When Jerry was just a youngster he would instinctively place his hands on someone who was hurting. It was how he tried to help with the simple approach so common to a child – he had no inhibitions. But after being scolded repeatedly for touching people who didn't want to be touched, Jerry was taught that unwanted touching just wasn't appropriate behavior.

Jerry also learned that if he touched someone he got a lot more information than he needed for a healing. If he put his hands on someone, it became very uncomfortable for him. Because he didn't just see what was physically wrong with the person, he got everything about who they were. And as of yet, he didn't know how to turn it off, or even slow it down. Jerry likes to compare the phenomenon to the TV show, "The Dead Zone," where the main character touches someone and learns all there is to know about that person, even their future. That's how it was with Jerry, and it was mind blowing for him. He didn't like it.

But this time, Jerry's client was insistent.

"That's not how you're supposed to do it," she said. She then grabbed Jerry's right hand and placed it on her abdomen. "Now, fix it."

Jerry was a bit startled, but resisted the urge to pull his hands back.

As soon as she touched Jerry's hand, a flood of information burst into Jerry's mind.

Jerry took a deep breath and tried to control the rush of images, fears, beliefs and doubts. He also saw the cancer that was killing her. He saw it all. He saw everything about it, even what was causing it. He saw everything in an instant.

Eyes closed, Jerry told her, "All right. I'll just get rid of it."

Jerry then did what he calls a force focus. "However you call it," he explained to his hosts, "I put energy right in there, and just grabbed a hold of the energy, and just encapsulated it. Then it just floated away. The cancer wasn't attached to anything." It's how Jerry had removed cancerous tumors in the past. By separating it from its energy supply, the hope was the cancer would die on its own.

All during this procedure, Jerry's client was making strange sounds, like she's having painful cramps.

Jerry finished and pulled his hands away. "I'm really sorry," he said. "Was I pushing in too hard?"

She looked almost relieved. "No, no," she said, "I just had all these bad cramps and started feeling sick."

"Is there anything else I can do?" asked Jerry.

"No, no I'm fine. I'll be okay," she said as she pushed Jerry aside and made her way to a nearby lounge chair.

Within a half hour she was gone and not feeling well at all. "I really felt bad for her," Jerry explained to his hosts who had witnessed the healing. "I didn't know what else I could do. I think I really shocked her. She was disturbed by it, and she wasn't sure what was happening."

The next day, Jerry was getting ready to head off to the airport for his flight home, when he got a call from the tall woman's doctor. The cramps had gotten worse and during the night she had been taken to the hospital. While in the hospital she started passing a black tar-like substance as though she were having a period. On and on it went, this bloody black tar coming out. Doctors were worried, and they wanted to take her to emergency surgery to find out what was happening. But she said no, you're not cutting me. So they waited. By morning they had to sedate her because the cramps were so terrible.

Jerry didn't know what to say. He felt terrible as the doctor went on telling him everything that had happened.

But then later, the doctor said, a lab analysis of the tar-like substance coming out of her said it was cancer. They just examined her and couldn't find any sign of cancer in her body. It was gone. She would remain in the hospital for a few days, but according to the doctor, it looked like she was going to be just fine.

The doctor explained to Jerry that he wanted him to know that what happened last night had set his medical world on end. He said to Jerry, "You've just completely done something that is beyond anyone's understanding."

A few days later Jerry got a phone call from her.

"Jerry, I'm feeling wonderful, and I don't know how to thank you." She said not only was she feeling wonderful but that her sex drive had returned. "I've started having periods again, can you believe it? I'm fifty-five years old, and I feel like a young woman again! I thought I was over all that, and now look what you've done," she said to Jerry as she laughed over the phone. "I also owe you my life, thank you."

It was shortly after that healing that Jerry decided it was time to try to help more people. The whole episode had given him a sense of confidence that he didn't have before. He'd worked on some people and had good success. But actually putting his hands on someone was no longer something he was uncomfortable with. Now he had another tool in his healer's toolbox.

The next person Jerry met to help him on his road to discovery was Jan Ross. She owned and operated "Jan Ross New Age Books and Gifts" in Phoenix, and was a gifted intuitive and psychic, according to Jerry. She validated many of Jerry's experiences, and gave him more information about himself than anyone could know.

It wasn't quite an accident that the two met. Jerry had combined his electronic knowledge and artistic side to come up with jewelry he called The Guardian Crystals. "I met her as a result of a referral from a friend," Jerry said. "I had made up some small jewelry pieces that ended up being quite successful for a time. It was a crystal pendent that lights up but doesn't use a light bulb. It used a small light emitting diode. That was put in there with some batteries, and it lit up the crystal. It caught on, and I ended up making up a bunch of them because someone placed a large order. But they never showed up." With an extra supply of Guardian Crystal necklaces on hand a friend referred Jerry to Jan Ross because she sold stuff like that at her Phoenix store.

"Well," Jerry said, "they weren't cheap to make. They were solid silver and a lot of workmanship went into it. I went over. It was the first time I ever met Jan in my life. She was a tall woman, six-feet-one, and there is just a presence about her of authority. I was a little intimidated because I wasn't sure what I was picking up on."

But Jan loved the necklaces, and ended up buying all thirty that Jerry had. She was crazy about them. Jerry and Jan became good friends after that. Jerry and his wife would occasionally go over to her store to visit or have dinner with Jan and her husband at their home.

They both smoked. If somebody came into her store and complained that Jan and Jerry were smoking, she would tell them to get the hell out of the store if they didn't like it.

Jan Ross was a major force in Jerry's decision to move forward as a healer. In fact, the first person Jerry worked on while he lived in Phoenix was someone Jan knew.

The woman Jan sent him to see was being eaten alive by cancer. After Jerry worked on her, she had nothing wrong with her. Not even any scars from the surgery she had had. For Jerry, it was a good start.

After that healing, Jan told him, "There. You have your validation. You've seen what you can do. Now you have to see what you have learned from it." She told Jerry he wasn't fulfilling his obligations to God, that he needed to get on with it.

Jan was also constantly giving Jerry books. After all, she owned a bookstore. Jerry read book after book after book on all types of metaphysical and supernatural themes.

She would also give Jerry psychic readings. He would go over to her house after dinner and have a cup of coffee. Then out of the blue she would give Jerry a psychic reading. Jerry always sat there listening intensely for a couple of hours…and she would go on and on. It wasn't always about Jerry. There would be other people involved in Jan's reading as well.

Jan Ross gave Jerry greater insight into his abilities as a healer, and continued to push and prod Jerry into doing more. "It wasn't any lackluster effort on her part," Jerry said.

Jan told him, "You've got these gifts. You can do this. What the Hell is wrong with you?" Another time she said, "Jerry, you have this going for you, and you are doing nothing with it. You are wasting your time. It's time by God for you to do something, so get off your ass and go do it."

Jerry believes Jan was the one most responsible for his transition to healing people more often.

But Jerry was still worried about what people might think of him. According to Jerry, "Jan told me that if somebody says that I'm full of shit, then just tell them you don't care what the Hell they think. She was blunt like that. She just said, tell them to fuck off."

Jan Ross died in 2004. But it wasn't the last time Jerry heard from her. One night two years after Jan's death, she came to see him.

Jerry could always connect with the other side and sometimes received messages from dead people. Dead relatives or loved ones of those he was about to heal in a day or two would show up early, and suddenly, to explain exactly what was wrong with the people Jerry was going to work on. These kinds of visitations really freaked Jerry out, and he hated it when they came in the middle of the night. But Jan was a good friend. He thought it was good to see her.

Jerry was sound asleep.

"Wake up, wake up," said a female voice.

Jerry slowly came around. "Okay, okay. What?" Propping himself up with one arm, Jerry slowly opened his eyes and there was Jan Ross standing by his bed. Most people would be startled, or scared half to death. Not Jerry.

Jan said, "You have to go to the store today."

"Why?"

"Because you have to, that's all."

Jerry thought, yes, it was Jan, bossing him around again. Jan may have been dead, but her daughter Janet still ran the store, "Jan Ross New Age Books and Gifts."

"Okay," Jerry said as he closed his eyes and rolled over, going back to sleep.

A few hours later Jerry was struggling to get out of bed. He is not an early riser, nor a morning person. Jerry slowly got up and swung his feet from the bed to the floor. And standing there was Jan.

"Get up, come on," she said. "You have to go to the store today, remember?"

"Okay, okay," said Jerry as he slowly stood to get dressed.

Jerry eventually got himself together and drove over to the store on West Thunderbird Road in Phoenix.

When he got there, Jerry walked up to the sales clerk and asked if he could see Janet, Jan's daughter.

"She's not here today, but would you like me to call her for you?" the clerk asked. She knew who Jerry was.

"Thank you," Jerry said.

A few moments later, he was on the phone with Janet telling her about the visit he had from her mother. "Jan came to see me, and she was insistent that I come to the store today. Is everything okay with you?"

"Yes, everything is fine," Janet said. "I don't know why she called you in. I'll be down in about an hour."

"I don't know either." As Jerry was talking to Janet, he noticed a man nearby who seemed to be interested in what he was saying. He asked Janet about him.

"Oh, that's just Jim Watson. He's a psychic who comes in every Thursday for readings…but wait a minute, it's only Wednesday. Do you think Mother sent you there to see Jim?"

"Maybe," said Jerry. "I'll talk to him."

"Okay. See you in about an hour."

Jerry hung up the phone and walked up to Jim. "Hello, are you Jim Watson?"

"Yes," Jim said.

"I'm Jerry Wills. And I think I may be here to help you." Jerry explained what the phone call was about, and about the visit he had with Jan the night before. "Do you have any Infirmity? Is anything wrong with you?"

Jim had been listening to the conversation Jerry had with Janet over the phone, but still seemed startled when Jerry suggested he might be the one Jerry was there to see. "I have cancer. Or at least I did have," Jim said. "Thyroid cancer. I've had radiation and chemotherapy, but I've been wondering if it would come back. I've been asking for an answer."

"Would you like me to take a look?" Jerry asked.

"Sure," Jim said, who now hoped Jerry was the answer to a spiritual question he had been asking. Is the cancer gone?

Jerry and Jim took a seat, and Jerry prepared to take a look inside Jim to see what was going on. After a few minutes, Jerry told him the cancer was gone. It would not be coming back. Jerry did a little fine tuning to the work western medicine had done, repaired a few places where radiation and chemotherapy had done some damage. He knew Jim would be feeling better in a few days.

Jim said he wasn't surprised. "But I was happy that this man had taken the time to come in and follow his heart."

Jim, who was from Great Britain, had been conducting psychic readings for more than twenty years; and for the last three years every Thursday at Jan Ross' store. So, he knew Jan Ross before she died, and he wasn't surprised she sent Jerry to help him. "It was an example of her and him responding to someone else's needs," Jim said. To this day Jim's cancer has not returned.

Another person Jan Ross had sent Jerry to go see, while she was still alive, was Frank Baranowski. Frank was somewhat of a guru within the new age community of Phoenix, Arizona. He had a talk show on a local radio station that dealt with all kinds of strange and unexplained phenomenon like UFOs, psychics and channeling. Jan had called Frank once to tell him about Jerry and he was excited to meet him. But it was a couple of months before Jerry got around to calling him.

Frank wanted Jerry to come over right now, right then and there. So Jerry went over to his home in Mesa. Frank had a large office in a detached building behind his home. Jerry thought it made a great home office. It was warm and friendly inside, with lots of pictures of Frank and his guests on the wall. It was an impressive collection. And while Jerry was with Frank, they talked about all kinds of things.

Frank worked with different forms of hypnotherapies. His specialty was past life regressions, which was all the rage at the time. He had been featured on television programs such as "Sightings." He had also been featured in several books and magazine articles. He had become a celebrity with the Hollywood crowd, and to Jerry it seemed like Frank knew everyone. But Jerry had never heard of him before, and was really intrigued by what Frank had to say.

Frank told Jerry he was raised a Catholic, an Irish Catholic. But since he was a child he had seen visions and auras. It was not something his family cared to discuss because you had to be a saint to have such abilities. Frank was no saint. Frank said to Jerry once, "They tried to do an exorcism on me so I wouldn't see auras, and I finally figured out it would be best if I didn't talk about it that much."

As Frank aged, he decided he had to know more. So he started reading and studying everything he could lay his hands on. That's how he became such an expert. He became a sought after authority on everything considered paranormal. Baranowski was even teaching a course at Glendale Community College called "Pathways of Consciousness."

"He was the type of guy you could sit and talk to for hours, and he was always happy to see you," Jerry said. "He was always the same Frank no matter what was going on, even when he was dying. I was the last person on his radio talk show."

Frank had some sort of heart procedure done. Jerry wasn't sure what it was. After being released from the hospital one Saturday afternoon, he was back at the radio station for his weekly talk show later that night. Jerry was his guest. Jerry had just returned from the East Coast and had driven five days to get there in time. He arrived just before the show, and soon realized there was clearly something wrong with Frank, but he didn't know what at the time.

As Frank clearly struggled to go on with the show, Jerry and another guest took over the discussion. The other guest was Sandy Rossen, a psychic who had lived in Phoenix but had recently moved to Chicago. Sandy proved to be an amazing psychic, describing exactly what Jerry had been doing only a few days before.

Frank died shortly after that. Jerry tried to help him but as Jerry freely admits, his gifts don't work on everyone every time. It was Frank's time to go. But Frank had been important to Jerry's development. Like the others before him, Frank had been supportive and encouraged Jerry to develop his gifts.

But unlike Jan Ross, Frank had a kinder nature. To Jerry, he was like this little cherub. He was always smiling. He always had good things to say, and he always encouraged Jerry without a condescending tone.

The education of Jerry Wills continued. The experiences gave him a sense that his abilities were real for them, so why not everyone else? They were older than Jerry. They had gone through those steps. And those steps had worked for them.

Jerry knew they had had gone through their periods of self-doubt. They had gone through the ridicule from people who would not accept them for what they were. But then there were people who came in who were accepting. There were others who thought they were valuable. It gave Jerry a feeling that it was okay to be in this arena and do what he felt he could do.

Because Jerry was searching for answers, he wanted to attend a Ramtha session scheduled for Phoenix. The Ramtha School of Enlightenment is based on the channeling of the entity Ramtha, a 35,000 year old spirit-warrior who appeared in a woman's kitchen in Tacoma, Washington in 1977. Laugh if you will, but that woman, J. Z. Knight, began a movement that thousands of people follow. She's made millions of dollars performing as

Ramtha at seminars costing $1,000 per person. Her Ramtha School of Enlightenment and her sales of tapes, books and movies have brought in millions more. Knight has also displayed hypnotic powers, as normal people regularly obey her commands to spend hours blindfolded in a cold, muddy, dark maze so they can seek what Ramtha calls the "void at the center." Some sources claim between a thousand and thirteen hundred people live within a fifty mile radius of her school near Tacoma, and attend classes regularly.

When Ramtha came to Phoenix, Jerry had to see it. At the time, she was charging about six hundred dollars a person. Jerry had only five or six dollars in his pocket, but convinced her followers to let him in briefly to have a look.

"Look, I can see energy, and I want to see what I can see," Jerry said. They let him in, and here before a large crowd stood this little woman with her robe on, walking around, waving her hands, talking, and spewing all kinds cosmic wisdom. Jerry was fascinated.

To Jerry, it sounded a lot like what his guide M had been telling him. And he could see energy everywhere. He could see it, he could feel it. It was like standing next to a crashing ocean, wave after wave of energy poured over him from this tiny little speaker on stage. He was standing there wishing he had six hundred dollars because it was so astonishing. But Jerry knew it wouldn't be right to sneak in and stay. So after a few minutes he left.

Essentially all these friendships and experiences were leading Jerry deeper down the rabbit hole. They took Jerry on a journey of self discovery. It led him to a point where he could stand in front of people and without grimacing, say, "Here's what I can do for you, and here is why I think I can do it, and maybe I can help you to get there, too."

The opposite was also true. As Jerry once said, "If it doesn't work, I learned to feel okay about that, too. I learned not to take responsibility for another person's situation."

Whatever Jerry learned, it was a complicated time. He went through a lot of years trying to figure it all out. A lot of it became trial and error for Jerry, and there would be a little bit of both still to come.

Chapter Five
Death Was in the Room

His time had come. After the healing in Austin, Texas, Jerry had decided it was time to start helping people. Jerry still grappled with the idea of charging money for his services. To him, it still didn't feel right to do so. But he did start accepting donations for his services if the people he treated had the ability to pay. There were many more he treated for no payment at all.

It was on a Good Friday that he got a call from a woman who said her grandchild was deathly ill. Her grand daughter's name was Nancy.

"Can you come right away?" the grandmother asked. "The doctors don't think she has long to live. She has childhood leukemia."

"Well, I don't normally see people in hospitals," Jerry said. In fact, he never visited clients in a hospital; he considered them off limits. The fact was he wasn't sure how doctors and nurses would react to his presence – they might make him feel unwanted. "Are you sure it would be okay with her doctors?" Jerry asked.

"It doesn't matter what they think," the child's grandmother replied. "They've done all they can to help her. I want you there, and that's good enough."

"Okay," Jerry said. "I'll be there. What time?"

She told Jerry to be there by seven o'clock.

Jerry wondered how the woman had heard about him.

She said she heard about Jerry from a friend of a friend.

Word of mouth – at this juncture in his healing career that's the way people found out about Jerry - if they knew anything about him at all. She also said she would pay Jerry if he could just come to see his granddaughter at the hospital that night.

"Now listen, Jerry," her grandmother said. "Nancy's parents will be there, too. They are separated, and they will soon be divorced. They don't get along very well," she added. "They might be a problem."

"Don't worry," Jerry said. "I'll take care of that."

"Nancy's condition started after they broke up," she told Jerry. "He lives in California now, while her mother still lives here. My husband, Nancy's grandfather, will be there, too."

"I'll see you tonight," Jerry reassured her.

The grandmother thanked Jerry and said goodbye.

After getting something to eat, Jerry headed over to the mid-town Phoenix, Arizona, hospital. It was Good Friday evening. He arrived slightly before seven o'clock and decided to take some time out. Jerry lit a cigarette, and sat back in his car, staring out the passenger side window. It was a still and starlit night, with not even a wisp of wind. The only sound was the nearby traffic, a constant rumble of car motors that Jerry often wished he could just tune out.

Thinking about the little girl, Jerry began praying for guidance and help. He still wasn't sure how the healing powers he manifested were brought into play. He had never been able to just will the inner fire that swept through him. But Jerry knew that somehow, each time he called upon it, his healing powers simply burst forth on their own, searing his inner senses with heat. Both stimulating and painful, it always felt to Jerry as if he had been filled with hot oil. Combined with an electrical current flowing through his body, it often left Jerry feeling dizzy with a sense of life he could never really describe to anyone else. This is what awaited him, Jerry knew, if he was going to be successful in his desire to help Nancy.

A few minutes later, Jerry stepped out of his car. He crushed out his cigarette on the black asphalt and blew one final cloud of smoke into the cool night air. He watched it floating past a streetlight and eventually vanish from view. He thought for a moment the smoke looked like a lost soul, a homeless spirit wandering the night.

Walking into the hospital, Jerry immediately felt uneasy. But a kind woman behind the information desk gave him directions to the children's ICU. His short walk down the corridor to the waiting elevators felt surrealistic. The only sounds he heard were the flop of his sandals and the eventual ding of the elevator as it arrived to carry him to the fourth floor.

Jerry had never been to a hospital to work on someone before. He didn't like anything about them. And this hospital was no different. Jerry knew what to expect: A full range of sensory experiences, the smell, the vibe, which was uniquely obvious and predictable.

The elevator opened to a large round area filled with doctors and nurses. It took a Herculean effort for Jerry just to step off the elevator and into the children's ICU. He watched as assistants carried medical equipment to and fro. Medical charts hung in neat rows at one end of the large circular nurses station in the center of the room. A computer monitor illuminated the face of a tired looking man Jerry later would discover was Nancy's doctor. Nearby, a nurse wrote notes on a chart and hung it at the end of a long row of charts already in place. A male nurse stepped into the elevator Jerry had just walked out of.

Taking a few more steps into the room, Jerry looked at the room numbers in front of him, and quickly determined that Nancy's room would be to his left. Not wanting someone to walk up and ask why he was there, Jerry quickly moved down the corridor of patient rooms.

Now about fifteen minutes late, Jerry was a little embarrassed as he pushed open the already slightly opened door to Nancy's room. He knew the family members had been there for who knows how long, especially after being told that nothing else could be done for the child and granddaughter.

As Jerry looked around the room, meeting the gaze of family members, he immediately felt their sorrow. The depth and gravity of the situation could be seen in each of their tired and tear streaked faces. Modern medicine had played itself out. Nothing had worked. All conventional options were exhausted. The desperation in their eyes was something Jerry had seen before, but never this intense.

"Sorry I'm late," Jerry said as he walked in. "I'm here to see Nancy."

Each family member introduced him or herself. As Nancy's grandmother had promised, she was there along with her husband, and Nancy's mother and father.

Jerry was surprised to see how small and cluttered the room seemed to be. Monitors beeped and whirred, bright displays indicated their functions, of which Jerry had no clue. The room was a pale blue, illuminated with bright fluorescent lights recessed into the ceiling. A TV mounted on the wall was off.

Jerry also noticed a slight medicine smell in the air-conditioned hospital chill. Balloons floated in clusters at the foot of Nancy's bed. "Get Well Soon" was written upon each one, suggesting the hope they intended to convey should she ever again open her eyes long enough to read them.

Jerry could also smell the sweetness of an arrangement of flowers that sat by themselves upon a small table with a small card carrying a similar message. Stuffed animals also adorned the side of Nancy's bed and other places of honor around her room. Their happy smiling faces and bright ribbons warmed the otherwise sterile hospital environment. Clearly, thought Jerry, this is a child who is loved.

Each person in the room stood on the left side of Nancy's bed. Her mother was at her side, gently stroking her daughter's head, and her remaining small wisps of blond hair. Nancy's father stood a foot away with a grave look that seemed to be cast beyond Jerry as he looked in his direction.

After introducing himself, each person in the room gave Jerry a different portion of Nancy's story.

"She had suddenly gotten sick," said her mother. "Tests were performed, and a severe form of childhood leukemia was diagnosed."

"Chemotherapy had been tried," said Nancy's grandmother, "without success."

"They even tried bone marrow transplants," the father said. But that hadn't worked either.

As he stood over the child who looked deathly ill, Jerry pulled a small trinket from his pocket. It was a little gold ball that made a jingling sound when he shook it. It had been a gift after working on a woman in Germany. Jerry considered it a good luck charm. After taking one look at the girl, he thought he might need it. "I knew I had it for a reason but I didn't know why."

The eight-year-old girl lay still on the bed before him. She lay motionless upon a clean set of blue hospital sheets. Her pretty face was turned slightly to one side as if in a deep sleep. It was almost impossible to tell if she was breathing unless Jerry carefully watched her small chest gently rise and fall.

An exposed arm revealed catheters, surgical needles piercing delicate skin in a vain attempt to keep her hydrated, medicated and alive.

A feeding tube had been inserted into the collarbone area of her neck. Jerry could see residue from her last meal still clinging to the inner pathway of the tube. The incision looked inflamed and sore.

"She's been in so much pain, they've been giving her morphine," Nancy's mother said. "She's now at a level they consider dangerous. The doctors told us…well, they don't expect her to wake up." She could barely get the words out.

Looking down at the little girl again, Jerry thought it was one of the saddest things he had ever seen. She just lay there so lifeless.

"She hasn't been able to sleep at all during the night," her mother said regaining a measure of composure. "She's been in so much pain. And it's been this way for a couple of weeks."

Emotions were thick in the small room, something Jerry had expected. He was a sponge soaking up every emotional detail, a common occurrence as Jerry prepared to work with someone. He had figured out long ago it was necessary if he were going to fully connect with others he wanted to help. He wanted to know why the illness had happened and if it was part of God's plan. Allowing himself to absorb the emotions gave him small and large pieces of the puzzle he would need in order to help.

Suddenly, as if a switch had been thrown, Jerry felt a deep calm and sense of purpose come over him. The coolness of the room was no longer noticeable. More and more heat moved through his body and down through his arms to his hands which now felt hot. It felt as if he had suddenly moved from shadow to full summer sunlight. A slight tingle of electricity ran through his hands, and there was a great rush of energy Jerry felt deep within his midsection, rising up to his chest and through his spine. It began to alter his vision and his senses.

As Jerry looked at the girl in more detail, colors migrated near her body. He had always seen these colors and shapes, their strength and tint told him the condition of his client. Strong and bright, the person was healthy. Dim and dark, the person was ill. There was very little strength or vibrancy in the colors around Nancy.

Jerry reached out and touched Nancy's small hand. Immediately, he received a rush of

information. The room no longer existed for Jerry.
Instead he was somewhere deep within the girl's
memories. As was always the case for Jerry, he
could touch a person and see their story. It helped
him assemble a more complete picture of their life
and what had happened to make them ill. As Jerry
looked deeper into Nancy's memory, he could see
the faces and hear the voices of her parents
screaming at each other. He felt Nancy's anguish at
her parents' seemingly endless fights.

Jerry released the girl's hand and looked at
each parent. He didn't want to judge them; that was
not why he was there. He only wanted to help. But
he knew without their cooperation, he would not be
able to help their daughter.

"You must understand," Jerry began, "that
love is the innate power of God. It is because of
love all things are possible." Focusing more on the
parents, Jerry said, "I need your help. I need you to
put aside your differences and once again love each
other. Love is not judgmental. It simply exists as a
state of being. If you can do this, my work will be
enhanced. Your love created her and from what I
can see," Jerry said, "your absence of love is killing
her."

Nancy's parents seemed ashamed as they
looked hopelessly at the floor by Nancy's bed.

But Jerry didn't let up. "To her, you are the
creator. If you want to help, it must be provided
through your love."

Now startled by what Jerry said, Nancy's parents looked at each other and immediately agreed to whatever was necessary.

"Whatever you say," she said.

The father nodded in agreement.

Jerry thought of something that might help. "Try to remember the time when you fell in love, and love each other like that now. Feel those same feelings. Do it now," Jerry said quite firmly as he pointed at the couple. "Do it now for her life is at stake."

The former husband and wife again nodded in agreement. Holding hands and softly sobbing, they lowered their heads as if in prayer.

Jerry now walked to the door, and shut it. Then he said, "I request that we not be disturbed."

He walked slowly back to Nancy's bedside, but with a sense of weightlessness. 'Could I help?' he wondered. He never knew for sure what the outcome might be. Experience taught him it was never in his power to know. He had to disconnect from the past and hope for the best. Sometimes he simply showed up, and things happened. Sometimes they were miraculous things. All he could do was remain confident of what he was and what he could do. The rest was in God's hands.

But this was no ordinary case. The sight of the sick child before him had a profound effect. Jerry had never really seen anyone like that, especially a child. He felt a hurt inside that this little girl was suffering so much. Right then and there, he decided that it couldn't be this way.

For Jerry the whole thing was very sad, but he slowly came to realize that sadness was not the only emotion he was experiencing. He was feeling something beyond that. He was upset over what had happened to the girl. No, he wasn't just upset, he was angry. Clearly, death was in the room. He had to do something to stop it.

As the emotions continued to bubble up inside Jerry, he turned to face the grandmother and grandfather. "Whatever you do," Jerry said, "do not break your concentration. Keep breathing. Keep praying." They, too, said yes. Everyone in the room now said they would do their part. And Jerry wasn't just asking – he was commanding.

Jerry walked up closer to the child. He looked down into her eyes. They were half opened, and she looked at him in a drug-induced state. To Jerry, she seemed to be asking, "Who are you?"

"Hello there," Jerry said. "Think of me as an angel with some music." He took a hold of the little golden ball he carried, and shook it in front of her. It made its little tinkling sound. To Jerry it sounded like a music box without any notes, just a series of sweet sounds. The little girl smiled and closed her eyes as if asleep.

It was time. Jerry began by running his hands a few inches above the girl's body through its slight and dying energy field. He knew the field would immediately respond to his presence, and it did. He also knew that if anything were to happen to help Nancy, it would be now.

As he moved his hand from her feet to her head, he maintained a keen awareness of what was going on within him. He could feel the changes. And after a second pass, he felt a stirring inside. The process had begun.

An inner feeling of heat and electricity surged and fell within each breath. He became aware of his heartbeat, his racing heart he had experienced moments before faded away until he couldn't feel his pulse. The air in the room was completely still. Silence seemed to have been created by the vacuum of energy moving through his body. It wasn't just quiet; it was silent.

Sweat began to break out on his forehead as his inner fire continued to burn. His hands felt as they were immersed in painfully hot water. Calm waves of heat and electricity washed through his body repeatedly. His mouth felt parched as if he had not drunk water in days. A mild shock jolted his body. Catching him off guard, Jerry looked up to see if anyone had noticed. He felt a little exposed. But no one seemed to notice.

Jerry's ability to see inside the girl was now fully engaged. Looking inside he clearly saw her condition was indeed as grave as her family had suspected. Already informed that Nancy suffered from leukemia, Jerry went straight to the little girl's blood stream. Jerry's abilities to move his sight into and through the girl's body would be similar to

110

anyone else looking inside a fish tank, and then becoming one of the fish.

Swimming into Nancy's blood stream, Jerry narrowed his focus to the individual blood cells. He carefully examined everything he came into contact with while passing through tissue and membrane. Had she been exposed to something chemical or viral? It was too early to know with any certainty. Jerry needed more answers.

Jerry then attached his consciousness to a volume of blood as it surged past him, and then froze it in time. He had noticed something. Platelets, red and white blood cells, and a variety of other components filled the area of his attention. Each with its shape, luminous field and color told Jerry a story about its condition. But he also saw one of her greatest threats – yeast had somehow moved past the safeguards of her anatomy and into her blood supply. A variety of cells had mobilized to eliminate the threat. But because of her weakened condition her body was struggling to defend itself. The use of antibiotics had helped slightly, but her immune system had failed to restore itself from the repeated doses of chemotherapy.

To Jerry, the yeast appeared dull yellow from the use of antibiotics. There were also more bright yellow seeds of yeast with small brown bulging areas across their surface. Many of these yeast cells were bound together as if mutated. To get rid of it, Jerry needed to know where it had entered the girl's bloodstream.

Switching his attention, Jerry discovered the reason for Nancy's yeast blood infection. She had been fitted with a feeding tube that had been inserted through her collarbone and into her stomach. Here Jerry found several inflamed and bleeding areas. This was where yeast had entered her blood supply.

The tubes had even created two ulcers in the little girl's stomach.

Jerry now began to breathe slowly and deeply. It was how he collected his energy. Depending on the condition and volume of energy he needed, he might take several breaths. Once filled with energy, Jerry immediately noticed changes within his own body, the most noticeable were in his hands. With each breath they became hotter and hotter as he continued to collect and store energy. Then with another breath exhaled, Jerry released the energy into the area he was focused on. There were times when Jerry's own hand print was left on the body of someone he worked on, looking similar to sunburn. For Nancy, Jerry decided to keep his hands above her body to keep this from happening.

Within just a few minutes, the wound on Nancy's collarbone had closed and rapid healing was taking place. Her own immune system was attacking and killing the remaining yeast in her bloodstream.

The instance when she contracted leukemia had been Jerry's original objective. Having seen the infection and its causes was an unexpected side trip.

Jerry suspected that Nancy's leukemia was essentially the result of stress. He knew stress could weaken even the most healthy and strongest people. And as her body weakened, her system was unable to restore itself. Leukemia, Jerry knew, was a disease of the blood where the very essence of life ebbs away until all that is left is a vicious mixture of damaged and life-threatening blood cells.

Jerry knew it would be necessary to revisit the blood supply. Cells had been reprogrammed and a change was necessary to eliminate the disease.

Jerry quickly studied the shape and color of the damaged blood cells. Their nucleus was darker and the field surrounding these cells was dim. Their shape was malformed as if having been squeezed at the edges. Many were dead or dying, their broken membranes floating lifelessly through his view.

Jerry now directed his attention on the inner sanctums of the cell's nucleus. The fluid of the nucleus was distressed and toxic from the administered chemotherapy. Jerry had seen this before. But besides that, he now saw the disease.

Trying to adapt to the changes brought on by environmental toxins and emotional strain, the cells had become so weak that they changed their inner programming. One by one, cells weakened even further. Working overtime to keep the body clean of harmful or unnecessary contaminates, killer cells had been produced to eliminate the weak cells. Leukemia was the result.

Feeling he was now at the crux of the problem, Jerry shifted his attention to bring the cell's own DNA into view. At that point, Jerry knew that Nancy's body was still capable of manufacturing everything needed to cure her disease. Once the DNA in her cells responded to Jerry's energy, he coerced her body to create what was needed. Nancy was fortunate. It has not always been the case with someone so ill.

Jerry then moved on to Nancy's damaged liver and kidneys. The liver had been severely compromised by the rampaging yeast infection, and her kidneys had been unable to fight off infection.

There are times when something is so badly diseased that it becomes unusable. This was the case with Nancy's liver and kidneys. Jerry had to completely deconstruct the organs and then reform them.

It was not an easy thing to do. Providing the essential elements were there, and in this case they were, Jerry did not believe it was a violation of destiny. He typically uses his own body as a template, and if this does not do, he reconstructs the tissue based on how it was at an earlier time in his client's life. Jerry knew that these changes might take place as quickly as the blink of an eye, or take several days. It is usually based on Jerry's available energy levels, his state of concentration, and the individual. In this case, Jerry was so desperate to help Nancy that her organs reformed quickly, and began to function normally, immediately helping her system destroy remaining yeast and damaged blood cells.

This once perfectly healthy child had been on the verge of death. But Jerry now knew she would recover.

While all this was happening, Jerry and the others noticed the room was getting hotter and hotter. But the others dared not complain or say a word. They couldn't break their concentration. The parents kept thinking about the good times and love they shared. The grandparents kept praying and loving their grandchild. None of them moved an inch or said a word. No matter how uncomfortable the heat made them.

Sweat continued to drip off Jerry's face. His shirt was soaked. The room was hotter than it had ever been.

But as it had started, the energy flowing through Jerry now subsided. With each breath it lessened until a cool feeling on his face and hands became apparent. Now standing upright, Jerry released a slow breath and once again felt his own heart beating slowly.

But within a few seconds…things began to go wrong. He slowly became aware of his own condition. Dizzy and disoriented, Jerry struggled to walk to a nearby chair, but nearly collapsed to the floor. Nancy's father caught him on the way down, and helped him to the chair. Her mother brought Jerry a glass of water.

"Are you all right?" she asked.

"What happened?" the father asked. "Did you help her?"

The questions came fast and furious, but Jerry was too stunned to answer. The room was spinning, and Jerry felt weaker than he had ever remembered. He couldn't answer them.

"I need to leave the room," was all Jerry said. He struggled to his feet, and with two people holding him steady, he was guided out the now open door into the hallway.

One of the nurses came running up to Jerry. "Is everything okay? What happened in there?"

Nancy's grandmother said, "Yes, we're okay. Jerry just needs to sit down somewhere."

"What was going on in there?" the nurse asked. "I tried to get in, but the door was locked. I knocked and knocked but no one answered."

The four family members looked at each other with puzzled expressions. "We didn't hear you," Nancy's father said. "And there's no lock on the door."

The nurse walked away, clearly determined to check the door for herself. A moment later she returned. "You're right. There's no lock on the door."

Then she looked straight at Jerry. "How did you do that?"

"I didn't want to be disturbed," Jerry mumbled, still dazed and weakened by the experience.

"Let's take him over here," the nurse said as she helped them guide Jerry to a nurse's office close by.

Jerry finally sat and tried to clear his head. The lights were out in the room, and to Jerry the air felt cool and fresh. He eventually came to realize that it had to be the morphine circulating through Nancy's body that he had absorbed in an attempt to cleanse her of all drugs and toxins. The drugs were poisoning her. Without thinking about the consequences, Jerry had absorbed it all into his own body. Now drunk with morphine, he sat waiting for the effects to wear off.

The same thing had happened to every person Jerry worked on. The illness and medications left their body and entered his. Fortunately, the effects were only temporary, and quickly faded away. It would have been quicker this time, Jerry thought, if he could just have a cigarette. But there was no chance of that deep inside the hospital.

Nearly fifteen minutes passed while Jerry waited for the effects to wear off. The more serious the condition of the person Jerry worked on, the longer it took for him to recover. He expected to feel more normal at any moment, when he was approached by Nancy's grandmother.

"Jerry, what did you see?" she asked. "Is there any hope for her?"

Jerry could see the woman was frazzled, and desperate to believe that something, anything could save her granddaughter.

"I'm sorry about this," Jerry said. "The morphine in her system caused a reaction within me. It takes a few minutes for something like that to fade away. I'm still a bit groggy, but it's getting better."

Jerry still tried to shake the cobwebs clouding his mind, but he did his best to explain what was happening. The entire session with Nancy had lasted thirty minutes, and Jerry was still exhausted from the experience.

He carefully explained to the four family members now gathered around him what he had seen.

"Nancy was very sick. She had stomach ulcers from the feeding tubes, which also caused a yeast infection. Her liver was damaged by the yeast in her blood. Her kidneys were overwhelmed by all the medication, and the chemo they used to treat her leukemia was a disaster causing all kinds of damage."

Every one of the people gathered around Jerry looked pale as death.

"But I fixed it. She'll be okay," Jerry said. "She has to sleep now. Leave her alone. Turn out the lights. You can sit here with her if you want, but don't make a sound. And don't touch her.

When the sun comes up you can wake her, but don't let anyone lay a hand on her: Doctors, nurses, no one. Understand?"

They all said yes.

Jerry knew that if another person's energy field entered the field Jerry had just created for the little girl, it would be disrupted. The changes Jerry made needed time to set – they always did. But this time Jerry wanted to make sure the little girl had a chance to heal.

"She never sleeps through the night," her grandmother said.

"She will tonight," Jerry promised.

"Will you tell her doctor what you just told us?" Nancy's suddenly relieved father asked.

"Certainly," Jerry said. He welcomed the opportunity. He wanted to be taken seriously by doctors, but he knew it would be a stretch for any medical professional. They were trained to look at facts and scientific data. The supernatural was not easily explained or understood by most people. Jerry knew that this doctor would have to venture well beyond the boundaries of his training if Jerry had any hope of being taken seriously.

But Jerry enjoyed a good challenge, and decided to give it a shot.

A few moments later, a doctor walked into the nurse's office, and Jerry introduced himself.

"You told those people their daughter wasn't going to live through the night, is that right?" Jerry asked him.

"I don't know about that," the doctor said. "But her situation is very critical. She could pass during the night, that's right. We have her sedated."

"Get the morphine out of her now," Jerry said.

"We can't do that," replied the doctor. "I don't know who the hell you think you are. You can't just come in here…"

The girl's mother interrupted. "Get that morphine out of her now," she said. "Or I'll take it out."

The doctor walked away and talked to some nearby nurses.

A few moments later he was back. "I think you are making a big mistake," he told the parents.

"This little girl had a really bad yeast infection in her blood," Jerry said.

"How did you know that?" asked the doctor, suddenly puzzled. "She does have an infection and an ulcer, and it has spread to her liver and is starting to damage all her vital organs."

"There's nothing wrong with her vital organs now," Jerry replied. "Just let her rest and tell the nurses to leave her alone. And as far as that ulcer in her stomach? There were actually two." Jerry told the doctor exactly where the ulcers were. "You have to get that feeding tube out of her but you can wait until tomorrow after she wakes up."

Now at least intrigued, the doctor asked, "What about the leukemia?"

"That was caused by emotional trauma," Jerry said. "It's been addressed and corrected, thanks to her family here. I fully expect Nancy to completely recover."

The doctor took a seat near Jerry and sat silently for a few minutes. Then he asked, "How did you know about the yeast?"

"I saw it," Jerry said.

"And the position and the number of ulcers?"

"I saw them, too."

"You know," the doctor said, "I haven't even told her parents about the ulcers, or the infection. How did you know?"

"Like I said," Jerry tried to explain, "I can see them. I can see what is going on inside her body, and then repair the damage."

The doctor seemed to quickly regain his senses, and walked out of the room.

After a few more minutes to make sure he was himself again, Jerry went back into Nancy's room and placed his hand on hers. A gentle, warm feeling immediately flowed down his arm towards her. Jerry felt sure once more that Nancy was going to be okay.

As he was leaving the room, Nancy's doctor walked in. Jerry leaned over as if to whisper in his ear, and said, "Get that morphine and feeding tube removed. She won't need it."

The next day Jerry got a call from Nancy's grandmother. "They checked her this morning," she said. "She didn't have a yeast infection. And she didn't have ulcers. She slept through the night for the first time in a couple of weeks. And when she woke up, she didn't have pain of any kind from that point forward…no pain at all! So they took out the feeding tube and she was eating and drinking on her own. Jerry, it's a miracle. We don't know how we can ever thank you."

Jerry went back to the hospital to see Nancy on Easter Sunday. When he got to her room, even he was shocked by the scene in front of him.

Nancy was already out of bed and dressed. Her grandmother was the only other person in the room, and she was just beaming at her granddaughter. Nancy was standing before a mirror wearing sweat pants and a loosely fitting sweater. She had wrapped a colorful scarf around her head, first one way and then the other, because it was cold outside.

"Hi, Jerry," Nancy said. "How do I look? I have to hurry. My mom and dad are coming soon, and I want to meet them downstairs."

"Hello yourself," Jerry replied. "You look fantastic." He was absolutely stunned. When he had left the hospital room two nights before, Nancy was unconscious and pale. Here now was a beautiful child full of life and excited to beat her family to the hospital entrance.

A few minutes later, they met Nancy's mother inside the hospital reception area. The little girl beamed with delight as she saw her mother.

"Hi, Mom," Nancy said. "Jerry came with me."

"Well, aren't we feeling better?" the mother declared as she swept her daughter off the floor.

"I don't know how to thank you," she said to Jerry. "You saved my daughter's life."

Nancy's grandmother took in the scene. Looking at Jerry she said, "We all thank you so much for all you've done."

Jerry just stood there and nodded. He couldn't think of anything to say. He was completely aware of the impact the change had on the family before him. Now they had hope for the months and years ahead. Somewhere inside he knew Nancy would be all right now and he could leave. It took a moment before Jerry even realized he had walked into a parking garage. Within a few moments, he was sitting in his car, lighting a cigarette for the drive home.

It was an important experience for Jerry. With God's help, he had confirmed a powerful new way to set things right. "It was all because her death was in the room," he would tell a friend several days later. "And it wasn't supposed to be this way. I just couldn't allow it to occur."

Nancy's hair eventually grew back, and the last time Jerry heard from the family, the eight-year-old girl had been enrolled in college.

The experience also helped Jerry learn to control awareness. Awareness is the best way Jerry describes his ability to focus and observe life around him. It also gave him the control he needed when he touched someone. Being aware of what was happening both outside and inside the person he was healing allowed him to block things he didn't need to see, to slowly examine what was happening to a person before taking corrective measures.

Jerry likes to say that he uses his awareness to slow things down, so that there isn't such a rush of information when he touches someone. Instead it's like a flow that he can regulate and comprehend. If he can't comprehend it, it's just a waste of his ability. The experience with Nancy and those that followed allowed him to slow things down so he could see even more details, and understand to even greater degrees why things happen or why things don't happen the way they should.

Jerry also knows the hectic pace of everyday life in the western world leaves him little choice. And it's the main reason people aren't as aware as they could be. "Moment to moment, day after day," Jerry said, "Our consciousness is overwhelmed with multiple points of focus. Being overwhelmed with multiple points of focus keeps us from being aware. Trying to do anything within this 'noise' is just another form of being anesthetized. Whether it's watching TV or listening to music or driving with the windows down, listening to the wind. These are all noises our awareness channels into us. It points our consciousness in a single direction. That's how we've learned to rest, and that's not always a good thing for us. To really rest you want to achieve an absence of thought, one "noiseless" direction for our consciousness to focus towards. With practice, you learn how to tune out the rest of the noise. Until you are able to do this, there isn't any silence."

An example cited by Jerry includes the simple act of breathing. "If you are breathing, you are not usually aware that you are breathing. You're just breathing. Your consciousness isn't there; it's on all these other things happening around you. But if you were consciously breathing all the time, you'd be consciously living all the time. Because breath is life. It doesn't matter if you are breathing the air in Phoenix, having a cigarette, or somewhere deep in the rain forest, or on top of a mountain. Being aware that you are alive brings life to you." Here is where Jerry believes that all the noise we live with every day can be a problem for us, and for him. "The things that you start missing out on because of all the noise, you lose from your life. As we lose more and more, we are left with a sense of emptiness, loneliness, desperation or anxiety."

It's one reason Jerry often escapes to the jungle of Peru or the deserts of the Southwest. "It isn't a process that takes a long time," he explains. "Come sit on a mountain top with me, or we can sit in the jungle. Or go by yourself, go out in the desert and just sit there." He says it takes a day or two, and that most people want the clarity that comes with peace of mind to happen a bit faster. "Most people don't want it in a day or two-- they want it in the next five minutes. Getting your mind to be perfectly clear and focused, that's the problem, and that's what takes time."

Staying focused and aware was important for Jerry. For if he were to continue his work as a healer, he would have to eventually get the word out. It was a friend who suggested he tell his story to a bigger audience. It required Jerry to take a leap of faith he wasn't sure he was ready for.

Chapter Six
Leap of Faith

Jerry was on one of his road trips, this time making a stop in Raleigh, North Carolina. A woman Jerry knew asked him to stop by a hospital in Raleigh and see a friend who had a brain tumor. Jerry went to the hospital right away to see her.

The woman was having another one of her frequent seizures when Jerry arrived. Her doctor, Stephen Banko, was really worried because he knew what the seizure could do. The woman's son was also in the room, and became anxious as his mother suddenly moaned, gasped for air and convulsed uncontrollably.

"Jerry, can you help my mother?" he asked.

"Yes, I can, "Jerry replied. He immediately took a deep breath and focused. With the woman beginning to convulse more forcefully, Jerry placed his hands on her head.

"I touched her head," Jerry later explained, "and looked inside to find why this was happening. I had already noticed the field surrounding her head, though I had no idea why it looked so odd. There were bright flashes and dark areas in this field. Small eddy currents of light moved rapidly. Once I touched her head I saw the blood supply had been interrupted due to a growth in her brain. The electricity flowing within the brain was disturbed to the point it affected the portion of her body that area was responsible for controlling. I changed it back to how it was supposed to be. Instantly, she was fine." The entire event took Jerry about thirty seconds.

The woman sat motionless and gazed at Jerry with a surprised look on her face.

The woman's seizure had stopped.

Dr. Banko looked at Jerry and said, "Oh, my God. She was having a seizure, and you just shut it off?"

Jerry said, "Yes. It wasn't good for her. It was going to hurt her."

"I don't understand," Banko said. "That never happens. No one can do that."

It was the beginning of an important friendship for Jerry. Stephen Banko would go on to witness more healings Jerry had accomplished. Each time he was amazed, later saying that Jerry was "The Man". "He's a good guy; no one should ever question his ability." Banko was so impressed that he would later fly to Phoenix every month from Raleigh to attend one of Jerry's healer classes and try to put some of Jerry's techniques to work to help some of his own patients.

Friendships are important to Jerry. Some of his closest friends used to work for an Arizona company called Village Labs. The lab was a special effects video and audio studio run by Jim Dilettoso. It had produced special effects for such movies as Titanic and a few others. But Dilettoso and his facility became most famous for some video work they had done on the Phoenix Lights UFO sightings on March 13, 1997. A UFO investigator in his own right, Dilettoso and Phoenix City Councilwoman Francis Barwood came under widespread criticism by the Phoenix media for taking the sightings seriously. Even though thousands of people from one end of Arizona to the other reported seeing several large craft, most of the newspapers and television stations in Phoenix never took it seriously, especially after the Air Force reported months later that the sightings were most likely the result of flares that were dropped by some National Guard A-10s over an Air Force range near Gila Bend. Never mind that the flares were dropped at least an hour after most of the sightings, most media outlets accepted the Air Force explanation and declared anyone who thought differently a quack.

Jerry had been interested in the work Jim and others were doing, and he became friends with many of them. They even formed a band called UFAUX, with Susan Gordon as their drummer. During their ten years together they played at special events across several States and in the valley. But as Dilettoso continued to attract negative publicity for his outspokenness about UFO's, the financial backing for Village Labs dried up, and most of the people who worked for Jim lost their jobs. Jerry and Dilettoso had a falling out over their personal relationship, and Jerry lost touch with him and most of the people who worked there.

But there was one man associated with Village Labs who wouldn't give up the fight, no matter how others reacted. His name was Tyler Pauley, and he was working closely with one of the producers at KSAZ-TV, FOX-10 News in Phoenix. Tyler persuaded that station to take a more serious look at the Phoenix Lights incident. The result was a series of investigative reports, which among other things uncovered an audio tape recording of an airman at Luke Air Force Base near Phoenix. The airman described how horrified several pilots were on the night of March 13, 1997, after they were given intercept missions over Phoenix. The FOX-10 News reports also included interviews with several eyewitnesses; even two Phoenix air traffic controllers were interviewed. They described what they saw flying over the skies of Phoenix that night, and said they were anything but flares.

Still, many other media outlets criticized the sightings as nothing more than out of control imaginations. One weekly newspaper, the New Times, went so far as to take pot shots at FOX-10 and Dilettoso for even exploring other possible explanations. The newspaper went on to question the techniques used to examine some of the video shot that night.

Through all this, however, Jerry remained interested in what was going on, and he stayed in touch with Tyler Pauley as Tyler continued to work with FOX-10 about UFO and other unexplained phenomena. FOX-10 had been the perfect outlet for stories such as these because the network was still airing a prime time program called "The X-Files", and producers were interested in anything they could produce for their newscasts that would keep viewers watching after "The X-Files" ended at nine o'clock. Tyler was the person who provided what they needed.

After months of producing these kinds of stories, which usually did very well in local TV ratings on the nights they aired, Tyler suggested to Jerry that he might want to consider doing a story with FOX. Jerry had seen the reports FOX-10 had done on the Phoenix Lights, and he knew they were taking these controversial subjects seriously. Unlike the New Times or other local media outlets, the TV station hadn't made fun of the UFO sightings or anything else Tyler had brought to their attention.

Besides, Tyler had been working for some time with Jerry and wanted to see Jerry succeed as a healer full time. He knew Jerry's gifts were legitimate, but unless you knew Jerry, or knew someone else who knew Jerry, you would not know about him or even consider an energy healer if you or a loved one were sick or dying. Tyler understood what a TV story about Jerry could do for his career as a healer. So after they discussed it, Jerry decided to take his own leap of faith. He decided that if Tyler recommended giving FOX-10 a try, then he would go along.

Jerry was very nervous about being interviewed. He was afraid mainstream television might ridicule him or attempt to call his efforts fraudulent. Jerry had full confidence in his abilities, but like many others, he didn't fully trust the media. However, after his discussions with Tyler, and seeing how FOX-10 had handled the Phoenix Lights story, Jerry thought it would be worth a try.

Tyler knew that all they needed was the right case. He had helped Jerry with many of his healing sessions, by hooking up Jerry with people who hadn't had success dealing with traditional doctors. Tyler knew what Jerry could do, but he also knew Jerry needed to be prodded along, especially with his organizational skills. Like other people who are extremely gifted in one area, they may fall short in another. Jerry is the first to admit he sometimes forgets things, and forgetting to help someone who needs it is not a plus. From time to time Tyler made sure Jerry was where he was supposed to be and when.

Shortly after discussing the possibility of taking his work public, Jerry ended up working on a man who was in very bad shape. In fact, doctors had given up on him.

His name was Steve, and by chance only, his wife knew Tyler. Steve had worked in the aerospace industry and somehow had become exposed to toxic chemicals. Neither knew the details. Steve had suffered some kind of stroke and had become comatose. The Phoenix hospital where he was being treated decided to move him to a terminal long-term care center. There was nothing more they could do for him.

"The place where they had moved him to," Steve's wife told Tyler, "was full of only two things. Old people and terminal cases. It's where they put Steve to die so he wouldn't be taking up hospital space. The doctors have thrown in the towel."

So in desperation, Steve's wife had called Tyler, asking if there were anything that could be done. Tyler immediately thought of Jerry, and Steve's wife decided to give him a try.

Hospital paperwork confirmed Steve's condition before seeing Jerry. He was admitted to a Phoenix area emergency room with a fever of 105 degrees. The report goes on to say, "He was found unresponsive...a CT brain scan revealed a right-sided frontal area of increased attenuation in the frontal temporal area without shift...a lumbar function was performed revealing cloudy yellow spinal fluid with a high opening pressure suggesting an infectious process within the spinal fluid, i.e., a meningitis."

It got worse from there. The report also stated that Steve "Neurologically was comatose." Steve remained on a respirator and "his papillary responses were asymmetric."

The report listed a host of related medical problems, including bacterial meningitis, a heart murmur, insulin-dependent diabetes, hypoxemia and Thrombocytopenia.

By the next day surgeons had given Steve a "right temporal lobectomy," and reported that "the remaining hospitalization was rocky at best…prognosis indeed seemed poor even at this point." Days later, the report concluded that "He had been in a coma more than seven days…so once again the prognosis was felt to be quite poor."

After that, Steve was transferred to a long term health care center.

When Jerry met Steve's wife, she told him her husband was going to be "unplugged," that the respirator was the only thing keeping him alive. Doctors said he was brain dead, and that she should start making funeral arrangements.

A day later, Jerry visited Steve at the health care center. Within a few minutes Jerry was standing next to Steve's bed side. Jerry drew in a deep breath and started by placing his hands a few inches above Steve's body. Jerry slowly moved from the top of Steve's head to his abdomen. Steve was in terrible condition. Vital energy centers were depleted and failing. The effort to keep him alive had only maintained his heart beat and breathing. Jerry saw that the energy field surrounding Steve was dim and still. Infections and blood clots had caused so much damage. As Jerry scanned into Steve's heart, it was clear to Jerry the doctors never expected Steve to come back because of his congestive heart failure. Jerry also saw that Steve's feeding tube was causing ulcerations in his stomach, and there was still a bad blood infection. "He was just laying there with his head on a pillow with several tubes exiting his head where a portion of Steve's skull had been removed," Jerry said. "There was no sound, no movement, nothing."

Steve's wife told Jerry she was running out of insurance money. "She had been told the best thing to do, the most humane thing to do, was to unplug him and let him expire."

Jerry had never worked on a client in such bad shape before. He didn't know what was going to happen, so he just started working on him.

"I started by addressing the head and brain area," Jerry said. "I took a long deep breath and extended my energy field from my hands to Steve's head. I was concerned to touch him due to the tubes and electronics attached to his head. So, I projected my field down and into Steve's head. Instantly I saw how the infection, stroke and blood clots had impaired the flow of energy through the brain. There was so much damage."

Jerry continued. "I worked on one small area and then another," he said. "The residue of infection in the brain had successfully been addressed by the medications Steve had been given. Still, tissue was inflamed and in shock. As I continued to work I sought to restore those areas and repair them as I saw the damage. Large blood clots began to evaporate, and blood flow was reestablished. My hands trembled as I worked. To be sure not to touch Steve, I occasionally opened my eyes as I sought the next area to work within. The field surrounding Steve's head slowly started to change, becoming more robust and luminous as it began to slowly rotate around his head. Within a few minutes it had surrounded Steve's head and shoulders."

Steve remained motionless and as if in a deep sleep.

"I moved to other parts of his body to reinforce the energy field," Jerry said. "Placing my hands above Steve's throat area and his abdomen, I focused into the field surrounding his body. Energy streamed into vital organs and filled Steve. I could see each organ as it responded to my attempt. One by one the organs became more illuminated. It was as if I were pouring light into a darkened place."

Then something caught Jerry's attention.

"While taking a momentary break from the deep focus I was in I felt a presence and decided to follow my intuition. I traveled deep into a darker, silent place. There, lying on what would appear to be floor was Steve curled up into a fetal position. I walked over, kneeled beside him and placed my hand on his left shoulder."

"Wake up, Steve, It's going to be all right now," Jerry said to him. "It's time to wake up. You're going to make it, Steve."

In his vision, Jerry saw Steve whole and uninjured. "He finally stirred and looked up at me with sleepy eyes," Jerry said. "I told him to follow me back."

"Your wife is waiting for you, Steve," Jerry said.

Suddenly the vision was gone. With a gasp Jerry opened his eyes and looked down at Steve lying on the bed.

"I was pretty disoriented for a moment or so," Jerry explained. "I hadn't ever had a vision like this before. It seemed so completely real that I leaned down and softly spoke the same words to Steve I had spoken in my vision."

"Steve, it's time to wake up..."

Steve's legs and arms moved ever so slightly. Within a minute Steve opened his eyes and moaned softly. It was clear Steve had awakened from his coma.

The whole place came unglued. Steve's wife started crying. Tyler pressed the call button to signal for help and the nurses came running into the room.

Jerry's friend Tyler just stood there and said, "I'll be damned."

Within minutes a doctor had arrived and the medical team surrounded Steve's bed. Jerry walked away toward the now open doorway and glanced back to the activity taking place. Steve's wife stood in the corner near the chair she had been curled up in. The blanket she had over her was lying in a heap on the floor. One by one the nurses and doctor glanced toward Jerry and then back to their patient.

Orders were being called out by the doctor as Jerry left the room. Tyler was right behind him as he walked down the dimly lit corridor leading to the parking lot.

Two weeks passed and Steve was awake and off his respirator. But he couldn't talk, and he seemed to be in pain.

Jerry received another call from Tyler and was asked to come back to work on Steve again.

"Once I arrived I placed my fingers on Steve's forehead and saw microscopic blood clots behind his eyes," Jerry said. "I asked him to close his eyes. Then I focused energy through my fingertips and dissolved them one by one."

Despite regaining consciousness, Steve still had part of his skull removed. There was a balloon-like structure where his scalp had been, and there were still drainage tubes coming out of it. Jerry thought he looked like a Borg (a reference to the Star-Trek television and movie series villains – a half man half machine race of cyborgs bent on assimilating humanity). Jerry thought it was freaky.

"I also found several tiny blood clots still lodged in Steve's brain. Each one seemed to vanish as I focused on them," Jerry said.

After spending about thirty minutes working on the blood clots in his brain and behind his eyes, Steve opened his eyes and looked around the room, then back at Jerry towering above him. There was a startled look on Steve's face, and he suddenly started to speak. He looked up at Jerry and said, "I can see! I can talk! Oh, my God... "

No one realized Steve had been blind. He couldn't see since waking up during Jerry's first visit, but wasn't able to tell anyone because he couldn't talk.

Steve turned his head and looked again at Jerry. "Who are you?" he asked.

"I'm Jerry Wills. How are you doing?"

"I've got a lot of pain, this terrible pain."

"Okay," Jerry said, "let's get rid of it. Where do you hurt?"

Jerry worked on Steve for a few more minutes.

"I saw the ulcerations in his stomach were the greatest cause of his discomfort," Jerry said. "The stomach wall looked red and inflamed. I decided the only quick fix would be to re-manifest tissue. I again focused energy into his abdomen. As I watched, the inflammation and ulceration vanished from my sight."

"My pain is gone," Steve said," but I still can't move my arms or legs."

"You still have blood clots there. Let's get rid of those, too," Jerry said.

Jerry looked into Steve's ravaged body, eliminating the blood clots. He also increased the energy flow throughout Steve's body and re-directed it to the troubled areas so he would feel better. Jerry again used his own body as a template to break down and reform parts of Steve's body.

Jerry said, "Okay, now move your arms."

Slowly, Steve moved his arms as his ability started coming back.

"Now move your hands. Make a fist," Jerry said.

Steve then started opening his hands and making a fist. He also started moving his legs up and down, jerking them around trying to get them moving again.

"Steve, you have a problem with your heart, and that's how all this started," Jerry said. "I'm going to fix your heart now. Close your eyes and relax."

Again, Jerry closed his eyes, and worked within the energy field enveloping Steve's heart.

"Steve's heart had taken a hard blow through this experience,' Jerry later explained. "Looking inside I saw the valves were weak and the heart muscle was failing. I believe this was because of toxic materials he had been exposed to for many years. To fix Steve's heart I had to absorb these materials into myself and regenerate Steve's heart muscle and its blood flow."

After a few minutes, Jerry was satisfied that Steve's blood flow and heart were now normal.

After this second visit by Jerry was complete, the improvements in Steve were startling to all who saw it. His doctor noted in Steve's medical summary that his patient had made a "remarkable recovery."

Within a week, Steve was home.

This was the case Tyler Pauley thought they could bring to the attention of FOX-10 News in Phoenix. After explaining the story to the FOX-10 News special projects producer, Rod Haberer (the author), Haberer assigned a reporter to meet Jerry and interview Steve, who was still in physical therapy – he was learning to walk again.

The reporter, with a shocked look on her face, returned to the newsroom after interviewing Steve and Jerry. Her eyes were wide as she came up to her producer and said, "This story is amazing; this guy is amazing. He saved this guy. I don't know how he saved him, but he did. It's a great story."

A few days later, her story ran on the 9:00 p.m. news at FOX-10. Jerry explained to a TV news audience that when he touched someone, he could see inside them and see what the problems were. The reporter described Jerry as someone who had power in his hands, the power to heal. Steve told the reporter he could feel the energy coming from Jerry's hands. Steve also said he was less of a skeptic now, because he was the product of a miracle. He also said he was doing pretty well for a guy doctors had given up on.

The story was a rating success, and the phones at FOX-10 News rang off the hook the next day. All kinds of people were calling to see if they could get in touch with Jerry. They wanted his services for themselves or other loved ones whom doctors could not help.

Anytime a news organization hits a home run with a story that connects with its viewers, it will not let go of it easily. FOX-10 later aired several other stories about Jerry, including one about Jerry treating another stroke victim, this one a young woman who was visiting from Poland. As the camera rolled tape, Jerry worked on the woman's left arm. The stroke had left it paralyzed. But after a few minutes the woman was able to move her arm up and down, and a big smile on her face showed how happy she was with the outcome. She could not yet speak nor walk easily, but she was clearly doing better after the few minutes she spent with Jerry. As with Steve and other severe cases, it can take several visits by Jerry to put a seriously ill or injured person on the road to recovery. The girl from Poland was no different.

Again, this story ran on the 9:00 p.m. news at FOX-10, and again the ratings were strong, and more people called the newsroom hoping to get in touch with Jerry. The two stories FOX produced were distributed by satellite feed to other FOX affiliate stations across the country and around the world. Many of them ran the stories about Jerry as well, and he started getting phone calls from across the country.

Thanks to Tyler Pauley, Jerry had received publicity he never could have received on his own. The FOX-10 News stories had been received well, and Jerry's calendar was filling up with healing cases. To make ends meet, Jerry still worked as an

142

electronics repairman at his small shop on North 7th Avenue in Phoenix. But more and more he was healing people. His leap of faith in a local TV news station had changed the equation. Jerry still had to be careful, and establish a new set of rules for himself about treating people. He also knew he would eventually have to settle on a base fee if he were going to continue his work. Jerry knew that charging for his "laying on of hands" would not be well received in some quarters. And it did eventually cost him some friendships. Still, he was now off and running. The Healer in him was in the spotlight now. There was no turning back.

Chapter Seven
The Healer

Jerry was now a well known healer. His coming out for the first time on commercial television was an eye-opening experience. Always wary of criticism or ridicule, Jerry had come through the experience mostly unscathed. He was ready for more.

So far we've examined Jerry's life and some of his early healing experiences. Before reading even more about the people he's helped, and reading about it through the client's own words, we need to take a time out and explore Jerry's healing ethics and abilities in more detail.

Jerry learned early on it would never do to just walk up to someone and start healing them. He always asks, and usually receives, permission before working on anyone. But surprisingly Jerry doesn't need permission to see what's happening with someone – that is unless he turns his filters on. Jerry sees energy fields around people – around everyone. He can see bright colors that may indicate any number of things. But as his abilities matured, Jerry learned to shut that ability off, especially with a large group of people. It was too overwhelming.

Jerry puts it this way: "I see energy fields around everyone. I see details around everyone, around people in a city or in a group or sometimes just people walking by the window. There is no reason to pay attention unless something catches my eye and I just get an inclination to do something. But typically, I just don't, because it is too much."

What kind of information does Jerry receive? He gets almost everything about a person's life. "Without paying attention, there is a lot of information that comes towards me," he says. "I hear their thoughts, sense their feelings, their emotions, their state of health and their state of being. I see all these colors around them, around their whole body, all in detail."

When Jerry does go to see someone, or someone asks Jerry to see them, the first step Jerry always takes is to ask for permission to see what is wrong with that person. "When I get permission to work with someone, they are aware and conscious and have given me permission, or they are unconscious and a family member gives me permission. If it is a child, the parents give me permission. Permission is a big thing with me. I will not violate free will."

Once Jerry has permission, the work begins. "It's in that moment that I drop my filters that I'm like a vacuum cleaner, and all the details are soaking into me. I'm like a sponge at that point."

Jerry begins by taking a deep breath, and as he exhales, the data stream between him and his client begins to flow. "I breathe in, and I breathe out. Within a few minutes, a few breaths really, I have acquired all this information. Now, I'm fully engaged. I can see everything I need to see around that person. I'm pulling in all kinds of details about them."

Jerry said at first he sees patterns around the body. Like the patterns a magnet makes when you hold it up under a paper full of iron filings or a pattern when you mix water with oil. He said the patterns are "as obvious as if a person has a big mole on the side of his face. It's obvious there is something there."

Jerry sees ribbons of energy running around and through a person. He sees variations running from one small area to the next that can signify something wrong, and the flow will guide Jerry in minute detail to the area that could be troubling his client. "If any of these colors are separated," he explained, "darkened or sharply striated into solid bands, I know a serious condition is present. Noticing where this band, separation or discoloration positions itself over the body provides clues about potential health issues. Examining this field is a first step to develop an understanding and nothing more. It is like opening a book and reading the chapter outline." Jerry can easily tell what the book is about from his observations. "Once I am satisfied with all I've seen, I alter my attention beyond the light, color and movement."

Now he's ready to proceed. Jerry will sit down and hold the person's hands or touch them. "The only reason that I sit down and take a person's hands is because I need to relax, or I need them to relax. But whether they're relaxed or not, it really doesn't matter to me. They can be all excitable and flipped out, but it doesn't matter. The important thing is that I need to be relaxed. It helps me do what I'm there to do."

Jerry sees a lot of people who are overcome by fear. He said, "They are just very afraid. They are told they are going to die. They are told a lot of upsetting things from doctors, family or friends. It's a very disturbing thing to have everyone discussing, asking questions, or treating you weird because you have serious problems. I can't get caught up in that. I have to be calm."

Sometimes, people are afraid just at the sight of seeing Jerry the first time. His six-foot-nine-inch frame can be intimidating, even frightening at first. But Jerry's soft and steady voice and demeanor usually do the trick, calming the person immediately.

As Jerry holds his or her hands, the moment where he really finds out what is going on inside that person begins. "The moment I touch a person," he said, "is really the moment that the most massive amount of information comes my way." And Jerry is ready to look more deeply into the body. "I usually move rapidly through these areas unless I feel a need to examine the skin or clothing. Clothing might contain residues of toxic materials."

At the same time, another set of filters kicks in. This time Jerry subconsciously blocks details about the client's life that Jerry doesn't need to know. "These filters," Jerry explained, "are specifically the result of not having any need to know private details of their life that they wouldn't want to share with anyone. I don't want to know their little secrets. I don't want to know any of that. It doesn't matter to me unless it contributes to me helping them. Everyone has skeletons in their closet, and it's none of my business. I never go there."

Instead, Jerry tries to focus only on their medical condition. "And I pull in all the details. It is really an emotional thing at that stage because I'm pulling in all the emotional aspects of those details as well. Once I understand the emotional connection to their condition, I filter out those aspects, too." Jerry begins to understand what the emotional aspect of their illness is, and a second filter kicks in to shield him from the emotional stress the person is feeling.

"Once I've got that, then I can see what's really going on. All this happens within the first minute that I touch someone. It can be ten seconds, it can be a minute, but it's usually not much more than a minute, unless I'm distracted."

As Jerry moves into the body, he begins to breathe even more slowly. Mentally, he enters an Alpha state and becomes very relaxed. It is essential for him to see with clarity, and to enable his intuitive abilities. Within moments he has quieted his mind, and he can begin to view the inner body.

Jerry is frequently asked what this "view" is like. "Skilled clairvoyants wonder if this is similar to their psychic impressions, where images fill the inner screen of their mind," Jerry said. "Those unfamiliar with such a thing ask if this is like watching a movie, or is it simply a feeling I get." But it's not something Jerry can easily explain. "Judging from my responses, my answer usually surprises those who ask. Most simply do not understand. What is it like? It's like suddenly finding yourself in the movie! Imagine that!"

Having now studied the shifting fields of color across the person's body, Jerry develops a theory of where to look more deeply. He said, "I follow the field into the body, attempting to find the source of the disturbance. Once I find this area or specific part, I decide to examine the area with greater perspective toward detail." For this reason, Jerry said he's developed an intellectual method to filter out, or filter in, aspects of the total view that's available to him. "I call these shifts of perspective, 'filters.' With this I can view details singularly or in various combinations."

Filtering also allows Jerry to view his client in different states of being. "Utilizing one filter and the body becomes transparent," Jerry said. "Now I see the organs and inner realms of the body. Bone, blood, arteries, muscle and each of the components are viewable, as are shape, color and workings."

Turning this view off and applying different filters, Jerry can see fields surrounding each, or all, of the areas affected. "Once I see where attention is needed, I focus myself in that direction and quickly arrive there."

Jerry's view is one suggesting he has become very small and has the ability to travel within the body. Remember the 1966 science fiction thriller, <u>Fantastic Voyage</u>, starring Stephen Boyd and Raquel Welch? The movie is about a team of scientists and their submarine-like vessel, shrunken and injected into the blood stream of a nearly assassinated diplomat. Their small size allows them to view problems within the man's body. It's not quite like that for Jerry. Instead of seeing inside a person's body like a movie on the big screen, he is actually there, and can scale his view as curiosity dictates.

Sometimes, Jerry will use his own body as a template to rebuild damaged tissue or a diseased organ. But sometimes he uses a different method. One might describe it as time travel. "Perhaps one of my most astonishing perspectives I access," Jerry said, "is the ability to seemingly move through time as I study the damaged area. With this I see how the item looked years past when it was healthy." How is this possible? Jerry said, "I work within a realm of pure energy, a locale where there is no distance or time. I call this a quantum field. It's where all energy originates, all matter manifests from and all things eventually flows back toward. This is a realm where thoughts can become manifest in our world if you know how to 'ping' the quantum field. From the perspective of you who observe me, it seems I work with light and my consciousness somehow focused. I knew as a child that light is the first ingredient composing the body. Light does not know time, and the quantum field from which light is a byproduct can be accessed to provide effects and material things in our version of reality, the place we call the material world. I help others by connecting my energy to this quantum field and directing it through my focus and intention. It's always been easy for me."

For Jerry, it is always important to understand how the condition originated if he is to repair it. "It is during this aspect of my inquiry I compel the story behind the condition to present itself," he explained. "To do this I have to move through time. In most cases this story is complete with sound and color. I experience emotions and each of the senses. There have been times when my eyes would tear from noxious fumes or chemical exposure, sneeze from dust or become very cold as I experience events with my client. The mind does not know the difference between real and imagined. My body responds as if it were happening to me in that moment."

The view of his client's life panorama is one where Jerry is immersed into a vivid dream. "Within this realm I slow down or speed up time at will to find and study events. I am determined to find any significant moment that might enable me to better understand, and further help my client." Jerry is never a participant on this stage, nor is he ever noticed. He is only an observer, living these events to understand the relationship to the issues he is asked to deal with. "This experience is as clear as looking at green fields through an open window."

Then it's time for the healing to begin. "Now I'm looking at the problem. It becomes illuminated and as transparent to me as looking into a fish tank. I can see details." As before, Jerry explained that whatever isn't working right inside the person's body lights up. And that is where his focus is directed. "Consider my view and experience this way: As opposed to just looking at a fish tank, I can put my fingers through the glass. It's kind of like having a flashlight on the fish tank and now I'm lighting things up. It's already lit up, but now I'm really lighting up specific things," Jerry explained. "And if I need to I can move in closer and magnify the details. I can go into it deeper and deeper and deeper, down to the cellular level."

Jerry's ability to search into the body at a cellular level is the key to his success as a healer. "There are times that I've gone as deep as individual blood cells or things that were tiny compared to blood cells." It isn't very often that Jerry has to do that, but that's the kind of magnification he is capable of. It's an unlimited magnification. "It's wild," he said. "It's in color, and it's highly detailed although some things aren't highly detailed, like nerve tissue. The more you bring it up, the more diffused it seems to become."

And sometimes Jerry must dig down into living tissue so deeply that he bypasses changes at the cellular level, and goes right to a person's DNA. It provides a fascinating experience for him as he enters that realm. "Floating as if weightless, long strands of bright fluorescence gracefully enter my frame of reference," he said. "Larger white pearlescent objects slide along the length like elevators ascending and descending in the colorful shimmering glow."

When Jerry sees just a single cell compromised, he knows it is a good indicator more cells within an area are damaged. In the event of blood, like with the little girl Nancy in a previous chapter, it can be alarming since blood must be in good condition to effectively deliver nutrients and remove waste. "I had seen numerous signs that Nancy's entire blood supply was compromised," Jerry said. "It was obvious her DNA had changed. This caused an unusual energy field around the cells, distorting the cell membranes."

Jerry said that DNA communicates with light. "Changes are holographic recordings in living tissue," he said. "As energy is released, field patterns change, altering the shape, color and function of a cell. These are the events responsible for the irregular shape of Nancy's cell membranes. At the core of all this is the shape of the field generated by the components of that cell, which is affected by the field given off by the DNA within the cell. If any aspect of a cell looks odd, it is probably due to the field being compromised at the genetic level."

Jerry said changes in just one cell's DNA are detected by other cells immediately. "The field surrounding every cell is like a series of patterns that all fit together. If one pattern should change, it upsets the harmonious balance throughout the body."

This is how Jerry identifies errant cells. "But does this automatically mean the cell is bad? Not at all," Jerry said. "If enough cells change within a short amount of time, attempts at modification are tried by other cells. After all, changes are sometimes necessary."

Sometimes too many cells have become damaged, and the body begins to destroy itself. "At this point," Jerry explained, "the proper instructions have become corrupted, similar to a corrupt computer program. In these instances, a backup copy of our DNA is needed. If the body is working correctly, a second set of instructions is referenced to see what is needed to recover." There is a reference still within the body's most secret places that Jerry calls "seed cells," which should not be mistaken for "stem cells."

Jerry said these seed cells "remain pure and unaltered our entire life, and are usually located in areas protected by the body against toxins." Places like the ovaries in women, and the testicles in men.

"Information about every aspect of our body is maintained within this biological library," Jerry said.

A complex set of checks and balances kick in once the body fails to find balance. "If seed cells are referenced, the following event is that stem cells are programmed with this information," according to Jerry. He says he can see the seed cells begin to glow brightly as this happens, and their light is received throughout the body. "Now programmed," Jerry said, "the stem cells locate the area requiring restructuring and begin to rebuild the body."

Jerry said that when this happens, DNA is fascinating and beautiful to observe. "Hundreds of differently shaped elements are woven together. At the end of each tapestry are small strings of material I believe to be useful as spare parts. The colors are at times neon-like and brilliant. Other times, the colors can appear dimmer, as does the luminosity. Depending on the health and function of the individual cell, these colors and shapes are different."

Shapes shift and fingers of light wave in the space surrounding DNA. Jerry says it is impossible to accurately describe, and more beautiful than anything he has ever seen. "The dance is ever moving and alive throughout the body."

But more often than not, Jerry does not need to go that deeply into someone's body. The problems are commonly more obvious to him right away.

For example, when Jerry sees a problem like scar tissue from an earlier accident, he clearly sees a rough tissue that is inhibiting the free movement of say an elbow or shoulder. "The ligaments and tendons connected to muscle or bone are surrounded by something else, like a sheath, and when it becomes damaged or irritated or agitated at some point, then it may actually kind of grow together or form like a cohesiveness where it isn't slippery and smooth anymore, but kind of rough." Jerry said it is the roughness and lack of cohesiveness which causes pain. "I just remove or smooth out the scar tissue, and the pain goes away."

In one case, Jerry described how he helped someone with severe knee pain. "I went in and there were dozens of these little strings around the knee where the problem was. One by one I followed it from in the upper part of the leg about ten inches above the knee all the way down around the left inside of the knee, on the left side of the right knee, and watched as he moved his legs." It's a good example of why Jerry so often asks a client to move certain body parts while he "observes" their function from the inside. "I could see how these things were not working right. So one by one I went through them and smoothed them out."

Jerry described how he fixes the problem. "At that point what I'm doing is basically de-materializing the tissue for an instant, and recreating it. It's almost like a magic eraser. If you ran this eraser over a picture you could erase all the lines on

157

the outside of the black line of the picture, like in a coloring book. You just erase all the stuff on the outside without any effort."

As Jerry changes the tissue, he says it dematerializes for an instant, and comes back the way it is supposed to. "In some cases," he said, "more often than not, the material that I've taken off is still there, but it's not connected. In the case of many people I work on, this material is now free floating. It's in there, and it makes kind of a crunching sound. Although the original problem is gone, there is just scar tissue floating around in there. The body will eventually reabsorb that and use it. Without knowing a better way to describe it, I implore this tissue to receive an energy signature that tells the body how to take it apart and how to return it back to other areas of the body to be recycled. Within a few minutes to a few days it all goes away."

In most cases, the crackling a person might feel in his knee is now gone. The tissue is smooth and fine.

"Saying that it's dematerialized is the only rational way I can explain it," Jerry explained "It's sort of a metaphor so that a mental image is generated. What actually happens is that the area is transformed into a field of living energy, reprogrammed and made solid again."

Jerry said it all goes back to his control of living energy. "Everything is made up of energy. It's energy first, matter second. Most everyone believes that they're made up of matter first and then energy, but that's not how it works. Being energy first is basically just the same thing as in any electric circuit." Remember, Jerry worked for years as an electronics technician, something that came so naturally he didn't even have to think about it. "You can take it apart, put it back together again, take the bad components out and the energy now flows through it like it should. Because things are made of energy they are also mutable as a result of the influence of energy upon them."

Jerry believes the only thing holding all this energy together inside each and every one of us is consciousness. "It isn't our awareness, but it is consciousness. Awareness is something totally different," Jerry explained. "We're not really aware of things going on in our body unless there is something wrong. But the consciousness of all creation is within, and flows between, cell to cell to cell. It's all being held together by consciousness, some greater force that I like to call God or the Creator. I don't know what it is, but it's what everyone and everything is made of, the creative force."

It's Jerry's ability to manipulate this creative force that gives him his skills as an energy healer. He explains it this way: "I compel it to shift into pure energy or energy that's being held now metaphorically between God's fingers. Then it is released and allowed to go back into matter again. And as this happens, tissue changes and it goes from being diseased into something that's brand new with nothing wrong… like there was never a problem with it."

Jerry cited another example, when he worked on Doug, a man with heart and circulatory problems. "When they checked him afterwards," Jerry explained, "they cancelled his surgery. There was nothing wrong with him. He had a heart of a twenty-year-old, no problems. The doctors couldn't explain it."

Jerry said the changes seem miraculous when he heals someone. And it seems impossible to all involved because it's so hard to understand. We don't have a model for it in our day to day life. We don't have a language for it in order to validate what is happening in a manner that speaks to the reality of the situation with any clarity. It's all done with metaphor and gesture.

So how does it work? In the best ability of Jerry to explain it, it's a combination of things that happen. "One of them," said Jerry "is a principle of physics that is yet to be understood well enough to effectively use it."

The other possibility is just as ambiguous according to Jerry. "It is the presence of what we are made of," Jerry said. "We are the elements of God, whatever God might be."

Chapter Eight
Case Studies

Several years ago, Jerry was in Raleigh, North Carolina, to treat a man with a potentially cancerous tumor on his pituitary gland, which is located in the center of the skull, just behind the bridge of the nose. It is about the size of a pea. An operation to remove it would require surgeons to go up through the nose, break through the skull and somehow get it out of there. The man who called Jerry for help wasn't looking forward to it, and like many people who see Jerry, he was open to alternative ways of treating it. But he was skeptical, only coming to see Jerry because someone else was paying for it.

"I don't expect any miracles," he told Jerry. "But my friend said you might be able to help me."

Jerry said, "All right, let's take a look."

The tumor was very aggressive, and had been growing larger for at least a year before Jerry saw him. Jerry noticed it right away.

"Do you want me to get rid of it?" Jerry asked.

"Yes, of course, if you can."

Jerry said the growth was really just a deformity. He later called it some wild thing that takes place when the energy within cells becomes distorted. So he just shut off the blood supply to it and directed the field to initiate a process causing the body to re-absorb it.

"All right," Jerry said to the man. "You shouldn't need anything else done. It should shrink and be completely gone within a week or so."

The man looked annoyed and said, "I'm having surgery on Thursday. I'm not canceling it." This was on a Monday.

Jerry said, "That's fine. I'll posture your nose and tissue to accommodate this. Even though you might be told the healing time will be quite long, I think you'll discover there will be very little discomfort. Your healing time will be a few days, not weeks."

"I conditioned the tissue to allow for the inevitable surgery this fellow was scheduled for. I placed a strong field that would remain after the surgery and preconditioned the tissue to rapidly repair itself after the surgery was completed.

Before Jerry left he told the man, "Make sure they do some kind of a test, or an x-ray or MRI before surgery."

"Why?" the man asked.

"You might want to make sure there's a reason to have the surgery."

The man said he would, then he and Jerry parted ways.

A few days later the man called back. Turns out, the man did what Jerry asked and had some new tests done. The results came in before his scheduled surgery. The tumor had shrunk to less

than the size of a pea, as if it were going away all on
its own. The doctors were alarmed to find it had
shrank. That isn't supposed to happen, so they still
wanted to do surgery. On Thursday morning they
removed what was left of the tumor. They
examined it and found it wasn't cancer, at least not
anymore. Whatever it had been, it was now
harmless, dead material.

Their patient was supposed to take about
two or three weeks to recover from the surgery,
which involved breaking into his skull through the
sinus cavity to enter his brain.

"I was told the bleeding should stop within a
couple of weeks, and the black eyes would slowly
fade," he told Jerry. "I was also told the pain would
subside in about six weeks. But I got out of bed the
next day, and there was nothing wrong with me. I
didn't even have the double black eyes! The doctors
couldn't explain that either, so they sent me home."

Jerry reminded him this had been set up
during the time they spent together during the
healing session, so he would heal really fast. And
he did. The doctors told him they'd never seen
anything like that before.

Jerry's client told his doctors he had seen
Jerry, and a few of them wanted to know more,
though none ever contacted him.

"The doctors couldn't explain it," Jerry said.
"They just said that God, or someone upstairs, must
be looking out for you…something like that. They
couldn't understand what happened. They had no

frame of reference for an event of this kind. Someday it will be as respected as any current form of medicine. That's one of the reasons I want to work with doctors. I think through me sharing what I can see and what I know it would allow for a mutual exchange of knowledge."

What Jerry sees everyday are doctors treating people as though they're the mechanic and the person is the vehicle that needs to be fixed. "You have a few screws and staples and if that doesn't work, you cut it out and throw it away. That's not a very good way of doing things," Jerry said. "You don't know what that's attached to. I had a kid I treated once who had a rod in his shin bone because they couldn't get the bone to heal properly. Getting the bone to heal properly is no big deal; you just have to know how."

It was April 24th, 2004. Ron Sissman and his wife Paige DeBell were driving to Fort Lauderdale, Florida, after attending a family funeral in Naples. Ron was driving his sister-in-law's 1998 Cadillac El Dorado to see his cousin. It was a Saturday afternoon, and they were driving along I-95 when someone in another car nearby decided to slow suddenly, apparently confused by the I-95 split to Miami.

Going about seventy miles per hour, Ron saw the other car, which was now going about twenty miles per hour, pull right in front of him. With traffic on both sides, Ron had nowhere to go, and despite hitting the brakes, his Cadillac slammed into the car in front of him. The result was a smashed-in Caddy with no steering. The car uncontrollably hit a nearby concrete barrier and then dodged across seven lanes of busy highway traffic – miraculously not hitting any other cars. Ron and Paige could do nothing but watch in horror as their smashed-in Caddy slammed into another concrete wall, this time in the freeway median, and shoot up into the air. It came down with a thud, and pieces of it littered the road. Ron would later find out at the emergency room that he suffered broken vertebrae and two ruptured disks in his back. Paige ended up under the dashboard of the car with a variety of bumps, bruises, and a wrenched neck. Both were also cut up badly from flying debris, including glass.

Emergency room doctors decided neither of them required immediate surgery or hospitalization. Ron's broken back was stable, and neither had life threatening injuries, so they were released. Without a car, and not knowing where to go, Ron asked the Emergency Room nurse if she had any recommendations. She said a nearby Westin Hotel on the outskirts of Fort Lauderdale was nice. So Ron called a cab, and they arrived at the hotel at about ten o'clock the same night.

Jerry Wills was dropped off at the same hotel at about the same time. He had been in Fort Lauderdale to help a woman who had requested his services. As Jerry was dropped off in front of the hotel, he noticed a taxi shuttle dropping off two people with all their bags. But he didn't pay much attention. He got his keys and went right up to his room. Once he was there, he just sat on his bed, thinking about how hungry he was.

Then all of a sudden, an old friend came through. It was Jerry's guide from the other side, M. M told Jerry, "Go get a Coke, you want a Coke. Go get a Coke."

But Jerry had just lit a cigarette and said back to M, "No, I don't want a Coke. I just want to sit the hell down, have a cigarette and watch CNN for a few minutes. I also want to call Kathy." Jerry then reached for the TV remote.

"Yes, you do," M said. "You want a Coke. Go get it now."

"What's this thing with the Coke? I don't want a Coke." But Jerry knew M would continue to pester him until he did what he said to do.

"Yes, you do. You want a Coke," M insisted again, as Jerry feared.

Jerry knew there was a Coke machine right outside his door, so he decided to get up and get a Coke, just so M would leave him alone. Jerry started looking for change so he could get a Coke. But all he had on him was a twenty dollar bill.

He walked out to the machine anyway, and to his dismay, it only took change or one dollar bills.

At this point, Jerry said to M, "I don't have any change. I don't want any change, and I don't want a Coke!"

"Go downstairs and get some change right now. You want a Coke," M said.

"All right," Jerry said. He went back into his room, put his sandals on and put out his cigarette. He then marched out the door in a huff.

Then he realized he left his key inside. Now he had to go take the elevator all the way down, get out of the elevator, get change and get another key to his room.

As Jerry stepped off the elevator and walked up to the hotel desk, he noticed the same two people he saw outside the hotel a few minutes before.

The guy looked at Jerry, and Jerry looked back. Jerry still didn't know this guy at all. To Jerry, he and his wife looked kind of beaten up and ragged. But he's in Florida, and who knows what has happened to them. Jerry then pulled out his twenty dollar bill and waited for the clerk. The clerk was still getting a room for the man and his wife.

"We don't have a car," the man said. He then turned to his wife and said, "Don't worry, honey. We'll figure something out."

The man again looked at Jerry.

Not wanting to be impolite Jerry said, "So, how's life?"

"Life's great."

It was then that Jerry noticed they both had hospital ID bracelets on.

"How are you doing?" the man asked Jerry.

"I haven't eaten all day. I'm tired. And I guess I want a Coke. I'm just trying to get some change." Jerry showed him the twenty dollar bill in his hand. "What happened to you guys?" Besides the hospital ID bracelets, Jerry had now seen several cuts and bruises on both of them. He'd figured out something must have gone wrong.

"We were driving down from Naples. We just attended a funeral for my sister's son who committed suicide," the man said. "We've just been in a car accident. I broke my back, and my wife has a neck injury."

"That figures," Jerry said. "I was told to come down here and get change for a Coke. But I think I'm here to help you." Jerry introduced himself and said he was an intuitive healer.

Ron Sissman introduced himself and his wife Paige.

Ron said he was interested by Jerry's offer. Both Ron and his wife Paige were open to some different things. He was a palm reader, who sometimes went by the stage name of The Amazing Ron.

After hearing Jerry's offer, the guy at the counter stopped writing.

Ron looked at Jerry again, and asked, "How much is this going to cost?"

168

Jerry said, "This isn't going to cost you anything. I was in town to help someone else, but now I think I'm here to help you, because sometime in the future you are going to do some great thing. That's why I'm here."

Jerry then said he could help with their injuries, including Ron's back and his arthritis. "I'm not here to put you on the spot," Jerry said. "Why don't you check in and go up to your room and relax awhile. I'll give you my room number, then you can think about it. If you want help, call me." Jerry then gave them his room number, and finally got change for his twenty from the clerk.

Ron and Paige looked at each other again. Ron was not sure what to say. He was kind of stunned. He thanked Jerry and said he might call.

Once they got to their room, Paige said to Ron, "You know, when he said he had to help you, he said he would fix your back and take care of your arthritis. The thing is," said Paige, "you never said to him that you had arthritis, and you didn't know you had arthritis until tonight."

While Ron and Paige were in the hospital, the doctors showed Ron x-rays and pointed out his broken vertebra and little spurs on his spine. That's the start of arthritis, they told him.

Ron told his wife about it later, but he never told Jerry. And he never even knew he had arthritis until earlier that night.

It was right then and there that they decided to call Jerry…mostly because they thought it was too weird. Ron turned to Paige and said, "Let's ask him to come up."

In the meantime, Jerry got a Pepsi. Turns out they were out of Cokes. Besides, Jerry now believed that M wasn't really sending him out to get a soda. He wanted Jerry to meet Ron and Paige, to give them an opportunity to let Jerry help them.

But now all Jerry could do was wait. He never forced himself on anyone. In order to do any good at all, his potential clients had to ask for help – had to want it. So, Jerry sat back on the bed in his hotel room, lit another cigarette, opened his can of Pepsi and turned on the TV.

Then he called his wife Kathy and told her what M had said, and about the people he met in the lobby.

"Who are these people?" Kathy asked.

"I haven't got a clue."

"When M tells you to do something, you should just go do it. Just listen to him, because there is usually some good reason for it," Kathy said.

They both knew it had happened in the past, and M was always right. "Yes, of course you are right. I should know better," Jerry said.

It was about eleven-thirty that night when Ron called Jerry's room.

For Ron and Paige, this is where the evening got interesting. According to Ron, he dialed Jerry's room number, room to room. "Jerry, it's Ron," he said. "It would be great if you could come up and help us."

Jerry said, "Okay, I'll be right down."

Ron hung up the phone, and took a couple of steps from the side of the bed. He told Paige, "Jerry is coming down to help us. " Then there was a knock at the door.

Later Ron said, "Now we could have been messed up by all the drugs they gave us or something, or maybe we just weren't paying attention to the time. But I swear there was like no time between when I called him and when he was at the door."

According to Jerry, he was exhausted when Ron called. "Now I'm like dead tired," Jerry said. "I've only had a few sips of my Pepsi, nothing to eat all day, and this guy on the phone says he'd like to take me up on my offer, if it's still open, if it's not too late. I pause a moment before answering, because I'm kind of tired."

Then all of a sudden, M decided to rejoin the conversation. "M says it's not too late, I should help them," Jerry said. "So I ask Ron what room he is in. And he tells me. So I go down, and we end up having this conversation for the next three hours. We talk about my life story, and we talk about his."

Ron told Jerry that his mother was a renowned psychic and palm reader in the New Jersey area for years. She was very well known, and kind of a wild Gypsy woman back in the fifties and sixties. Before she died, she taught Ron everything she knew about palm reading – she gave him books and materials she had kept hidden, and told Ron he had the gift. Now Ron said that he works sometimes as the Amazing Ron, taking free vacations to resorts in exchange for his palm readings for other guests. Paige, his wife, does body painting. She paints kids and adults, sometimes full body paintings. But now Ron was worried about their health. He told Jerry his back was broken, and her neck was wrenched, and that she was in a lot of pain.

Jerry went right to work. He worked on Ron's back for about thirty minutes. He found where it was broken.

"Yes," said Jerry, "It's broken all right...just about here." Jerry pointed to a spot on Ron's back.

Paige said, "Yes, that's right where the doctor said it was."

Ron pulled his shirt up and the doctor had put some magic marker dots on his back, where the break had been. And it was exactly where Jerry said it was.

"You've fractured two vertebrae, right on that spot," Jerry said. "Let me see what I can do."

Again Jerry used his skills to look inside Ron's back, and he found what it looked like at an earlier time, before Ron and Paige's accident. He then reformed the bones in Ron's back so they looked like they used to. The break was gone.

Then like Jerry usually does during a healing session with someone, he asked Ron to try it

172

out. "Ron, try to touch your toes," Jerry said. "Prove to yourself that what I've done has actually manifested."

"Okay," Ron said as he stood up and started bending his back this way and that. "It doesn't hurt, Paige," Ron said to his wife. "It feels pretty loose. I don't know about touching my toes though."

"Give it a try," Jerry said. "If it's still broken, you won't be able to, and it will hurt like hell."

Ron bent over and slowly put his fingertips on the floor, then moved his hands down even further. "Oh my God," Ron said. Then he turned up and twisted, popped his back and said, "Oh. That felt good." In an instant Ron seemed blown away by the whole experience. He had tears in his eyes.

Talking about the experience two years later, Ron remembered being wary about Jerry at first. "I've been trained in hypnosis myself," Ron said. "So I was looking for all the earmarks of being relaxed and being hypnotized to try to make me believe that I'm not in pain...that kind of thing."

It is a common criticism of intuitive healers that they are nothing more than hypnotists. Ron said he saw nothing in Jerry's treatment that led him to believe he was under hypnosis.

Besides going right to the spot where he had broken his back, Ron said Jerry worked quickly, too quickly to hypnotize someone. And Ron said he kept his eyes on his wife Paige the whole time. If he were being hypnotized, Ron knew Paige would spot it. She didn't see a thing that led her to believe her husband was under some sort of hypnotic spell.

And whatever Jerry was doing, Ron said it didn't last very long. "It was almost as fast as a person just sort of waving his hand over you. I don't know if it was a minute, two minutes, or less. It didn't seem like it was very long at all. He said I wouldn't be pain free right away because my muscles and tendons had been hyper-extended by the accident, and it might take a few days."

Ron also remembered Jerry asking him to move around and touch his toes. "I was sitting there when he asked me to stand up and touch my toes. I was worried because it felt like someone shoved a stick up my ass when I sat down. I couldn't get up and down into a chair because it hurt so bad."

But slowly, carefully, Ron stood. And he was pain free. "There was virtually no pain," Ron said. "I moved left and right, bent down like I was picking up a penny. I stood back up and looked at my wife. I said I can't explain it, but I don't feel pain anymore. It was gone."

Ron walked up to Jerry and gave him a big hug. "Oh, thank you, thank you. Now you've got to help my wife. She's hurt."

Paige came over to a chair near the bed.

She told Jerry she had seriously whip-lashed her neck, so Jerry started there. A few moments later, her neck pain was gone. But Jerry noticed

174

something else. "Paige," Jerry said. "You have a blood vessel in your head that is really weak. It could be a deadly serious situation for you."

Paige said, "You know, that runs in my family." Thinking she would soon die of the same ailment, she turned to Ron and said, "I know this is it."

"Listen," Jerry said. "This isn't going to happen to you. I'm going to fix it now. You are going to be fine. The headaches that you've had and all the dizziness that you've had will all be gone, and it won't come back."

Paige looked at Jerry and said, "I never told you I had headaches."

Ron asked, "How did you know she was dizzy?"

"I can see it," said Jerry. "Now, I'm going to fix it."

Moments later, Paige said it felt like the pressure in her head that she'd been feeling was gone.

Ron remembered being startled by what Jerry did to his wife. "When he worked on Paige," Ron said, "she felt the energy when he put his hands on her head. He didn't even start going down her body. He started on her head like he did with me and then he kind of moved his hands over her head. He had his eyes closed, and he was shaking his head no, like this is bad. Then he moved his hands to her shoulders, and told her he found a weakened vein in her head. He asked if she had headaches, and she said yes."

After that night, Ron said his wife's headaches never returned.

The three sat in Ron and Paige's hotel room for at least another two hours talking more about the kinds of experiences Jerry had while healing other people. Both Ron and Paige were amazed.

Before he left, Ron asked if there was one more thing he could do for them. "Paige gets this terrible poison ivy rash all the time, "Ron said. "Every time she gets near it she has to go to the doctors and they have to give her shots. Poison ivy is driving her crazy."

Jerry said he could take care of it. While Ron watched, Jerry put his hands on his wife's stomach, and moved his fingers in a clockwise direction like a thief trying to crack a combination safe.

Jerry said, "Well, I wouldn't go back and grab poison ivy. But I think I took care of it for you."

"That would be great," Paige said. "I hope this works."

It was some time later that Ron and Paige were doing some gardening. Paige had pulled a handful of weeds. But Ron noticed they were something else. "It turned out she grabbed a chuck of poison ivy, and had it all over her hand. That could have been death for her. I mean she gets sick from just breathing it, not touching it like that. But it turns out all she got was a little bump on her finger, and it went away. She used to get it all the time, but since we saw Jerry she doesn't get poison ivy, not severely anyway. It was just another little bonus he was able to do, I think."

In the fall of 2006, Jerry Wills was invited to Tamaqua, Pennsylvania, to see someone dying of cancer. The man paying his way lived in Phoenix, and his wife had just been treated successfully by Jerry for a hip problem. The cancer victim was his cousin, and he wanted to help. So Jerry received plane tickets and money to stay at a Bed & Breakfast in Tamaqua for a week.

Soon after his arrival in Tamaqua, Jerry saw the man who was diagnosed with terminal brain cancer. Unfortunately, Jerry soon discovered there was nothing he could do. The cancer was too advanced. As Jerry often says, he can't help everyone – only if it is part of their destiny can he help the sick or cure the injured. This man was beyond hope. The family asked if Jerry could at least ease his passing. "I can do that," Jerry said. He did a few things to help convince the man's body that his time had come. A couple of days after Jerry left he died peacefully in his sleep.

But word of Jerry's presence in Tamaqua quickly spread. The small Pennsylvania mining area wasn't a good place to keep secrets. A musician who lived in nearby Landingville also heard about Jerry from his friend in Phoenix – the same man who sent Jerry to Tamaqua in the first place. Jay Smar also knew the man who was dying of cancer. The three men had been friends for years.

Jay had been performing for more than thirty years, playing mostly guitars and other flat-picked instruments like the claw hammer banjo and various fiddles. (To hear some of his work, go to www.jaysmar.com).

Jay was also a runner, but after his second marathon Jay realized he had hurt something in his back. And unfortunately for Jay it was having an effect on his left hand. He was losing strength in it – meaning he was having trouble playing some notes of the many popular songs he performed. And Jay performed a lot. He could have up to thirty performances a month – and played worldwide, having completed tours in Scotland, Canada and most of the United States. His new and traditional brands of folk music can be found on recordings across the U.S. and Europe. Playing musical instruments for appreciative crowds was his life. But for six years, he was having more and more problems playing certain notes and some songs altogether. While not extremely painful, Jay felt a weakness in his hand that wasn't getting any better – not with physical therapy, not with steroid injections, or drugs. "I was still losing my grip in my left hand," Jay told his friends. He even tried one of those small balls, the ones with a loop where your thumb goes, and four more for your fingers.

It's used to extend your hand, to build hand strength. The ball helped Jay a little bit, but not enough. He also went to a chiropractor without much success.

So when Jay heard about Jerry Wills, he jumped at the chance to see him. Jay said, "When I found out Jerry was in Tamaqua, and my friend was paying to bring Jerry to come here for a week and stay at a B&B, and pay for his flight, I figured there must be something to this. It must be legitimate." Jay admitted such open attitudes aren't easy to come by in that part of the country. "I was a little hesitant about it, because here in the coal region, we just heard about the Beatles. This was like really far out, and it was a little mind boggling."

Still, Jay was excited to see him. "I thought this would be a great opportunity to visit this man, and not just for me," Jay said. "I thought about my fiancée who was having problems, her mother, and a friend of ours who has lung cancer."

But Jay went alone, not knowing what to expect. Meeting Jerry for the first time at a Bed & Breakfast in Tamaqua, Jay was startled by Jerry's size. "He is so big, when I looked up at him," Jay said. "He's like six-feet nine-inches, and it's like, Oh my God, it's very intimidating at first." However, like many others, Jay was immediately calmed by Jerry's demeanor. "I explained it later to my friends this way," Jay said. "In those old pictures of Jesus that we've all seen, I have some hanging up in my house, and there's a very calm look in his eyes. You just feel very at ease when you look at that picture. It is a very loving look. Jerry had that same look to me. It was just a very sincere type of look and a very peaceful type of look."

Like he always does, Jerry took Jay's hands and began his healing session. Jay thought it looked like Jerry was meditating. He also felt some light warmth from Jerry's hand when he touched his neck and back.

A few minutes later, Jerry told him his hand should be stronger... "And oh, by the way, you can run again," Jerry said. "Your back is okay now."

The most startling thing to Jay was that he had never mentioned that he was a runner, or that he had a back problem.

"Jerry, I never told you about my back, just my hand," Jay said. "And how did you know I was a runner?"

"I just know," Jerry said. "It's no big deal."

"Wow," Jay said.

"Just to check your hand," Jerry said, "can you play a song for me?" Jerry had asked Jay to bring his guitar with him. He wanted to see how well Jay could play after being treated.

Jay took his guitar and began playing "Nine Pound Hammer" by Merle Travis. He normally had trouble playing some of the chords, but not this time. His hand moved more freely to the right strings.

The results of the session, according to Jay, "My hand was much stronger, not completely healed, but definitely better."

What stood out even more was what happened to Jay immediately after seeing Jerry for the first time. "I remember going to the bathroom and washing my hands and feeling like something was happening. I just started to giggle, because I could not believe that this just happened."

Strange sensations continued during Jay's drive home. "I could feel something I can only describe as a spiral spinning in my neck, and above my shoulder where the original problem was," Jay said. "It was this sensation of something spiraling in there. It actually almost tickled in a way. It stopped, and then there was another one. There were two. It happened to me twice on the way home."

A couple of weeks after the session, Jay's hand was still getting stronger. Not completely healed, he said, but much better. "The same thing happened to two of the three people I took to see Jerry that week," he said.

One was a friend of his fiancée. She had been told she had terminal lung cancer, and was even more of a skeptic than Jay. "The thing is with this woman," Jay said, "it's her demeanor. She really has a crappy attitude towards everyone. She was an acquaintance of ours that we just sort of took in. We had to like this person whether or not we really did." A gracious act, considering the woman once tried to sue Jay's fiancée after she slipped and fell on some ice on her driveway. "This is a woman with a lot of negativity around her, but I was still hoping Jerry could help her," explained Jay.

But the visit didn't go well. "I don't think she accepted anything Jerry told her, because the first thing out of Jerry's mouth was, 'You have to change your attitude,'" Jay said. "And I didn't even tell Jerry about her demeanor or her attitude towards other people. The only thing I told him was that she had cancer, and that we were trying to help her."

Jerry picked up on the woman's negativity almost immediately. "Right off the bat," Jay said. "It was the first thing he said. I think that may have turned her off. That's the kind of woman she is."

Again, Jerry did his best, but with limited success, if any at all. "He did recommend she try some herbal medications, and I ordered some for her," Jay said. "We would just give her the money, but she would spend it all on gambling."

Jerry had better luck with Jay's fiancée and her mother. The 77-year-old mother-in-law to-be had a variety of problems, including dizzy spells that Jerry treated. Jay says they still occur, but not nearly as often.

Jay's fiancée Rachael had been warned about problems with her carotid artery, but Jerry checked it out and reassured her there was nothing wrong. It was a big relief for Rachael. He also fixed her back pain. She had a lot of trouble getting out of bed in the morning, but now she has very little pain most days, if any. "She can get up now, pain free," Jay said. "After that she told a couple of her friends, and they went to see Jerry, too. He was very busy that week he was here. A cat like that comes into town, you either believe in it or you don't."

Jay was just at the point where he would try anything to help. "I mean it was my career! I was literally at a point where I was re-writing and re-fingering songs I was playing for twenty years because I couldn't play them anymore," Jay said. "That's how bad it was getting. But now it seems like I have more strength and flexibility."

Jerry came home a week later, clearly exhausted. "I need a break," Jerry told Kathy. "But it was a very gratifying trip," he said. "We were able to help a lot of people."

As for Jay, he's very grateful Jerry was there. "I'm just glad that God brought him to the planet," Jay said. "We are very happy that he is here, that he is doing what he is doing."

Keli Aisaki and his brother were walking home late one night in southeast Phoenix. It was a cool night, February 24th, 2004. Keli was born on the South Pacific Island of Tonga, near American Samoa. His wife Josie was born in American Samoa, but is part Tongan. Both of their families moved to Phoenix where the couple met at church and later married. In fact, a small community of Tongan-Americans call Phoenix home, and most are considered members of the Tongan Catholic Community of Arizona.

On their walk home that night, four men confronted Keli and his brother. Some of them were Josie's relatives – and later blamed the whole thing on a family feud. However, most families settle their differences without swinging shovels and kicking steel toed boots. The four men viciously attacked Keli and his brother. Keli was beaten in the head repeatedly with a shovel. His brother was injured as well, but not as severely. When police arrived, they thought Keli was dead. His brother, in better shape, was immediately flown by helicopter to a local Phoenix hospital. Medics didn't think Keli would make it, so they took him by ground ambulance. There was apparently no sense in wasting expensive helicopter fuel on him.

Keli's wife Josie was one of the first to see him at the emergency room. She was told by doctors that her husband had been beaten so badly that they fractured every single bone in his face. Josie was horrified by what she saw. It looked like her husband's eyes were inside out. She could barely recognize him. His whole face was swollen and covered with blood. She only knew it was her husband by the tattoos on his arm.

His head smashed in by several blows with a shovel, Keli was not expected to live through the night. His doctors gave him a ten percent chance to live.

Josie said, "You are just in shock when something like that happens to a loved one. I didn't know what to say."

The doctors asked Josie to stay overnight. "They told me to stick around that evening in case I had to pull his breathing tube out. They put him on life support and they told me, look, chances are he's not going to make it tonight. So you have to stick around to unplug his life support."

Keli was completely unresponsive and comatose. Doctors told Josie that even if her husband did survive, he would have such severe brain damage that he would never fully recover, and never be the man he was. Josie, in shock, continued to take it all in as if in a deep fog. She didn't know what to say or do.

To make matters worse, hospital security and police said her husband may still be at risk from a reprisal attack. The four men who had attacked her husband and his brother were under arrest, but other members of their "family" could still try to kill Keli. The hospital set up a password system so only those who Josie approved directly could enter that part of the hospital to visit her husband.

One of the few visitors Josie approved to visit her husband for the next day was Jerry Wills. Jerry found out about Keli after getting a phone call from a friend who often sends Jerry to those who need his help but cannot pay for Jerry's services. To help these people, she pays his fee. Jerry was told that this man was hospitalized after being severely

beaten, and doctors had already asked his wife
about donating his organs. The woman had talked
to Josie about Jerry, and Josie told her she was
willing to give it a try. So at about noon the next
day, or six hours after Keli was admitted, Jerry
arrived at the hospital with his friend Tony Arnold.
After being cleared by security, Jerry met Josie in
the hospital lobby.

Still in shock over the condition of her
husband, Josie didn't know what to think when she
first saw Jerry.

Jerry and Tony introduced themselves, then
Jerry said, "I'm a friend of a friend, and that's how I
heard about Keli. And that's why I am here to help,
if you want it."

Josie thought it was weird. She stared up at
Jerry. She was thinking, who the heck is this?

But Josie was immediately disarmed by
Jerry's demeanor. She noticed an immediate
warmth about him. "You just kind of succumb to
him," she would say later. "So I'm like, oh, this is
a friend? He's got to be a friend, obviously. How
else would he know?"

Jerry again reassured Josie that a friend of
hers called him and asked him to come to the
hospital right away. "I wanted to come and pray
and see what I can do for your husband," Jerry said.

His words gave Josie a sense of calmness.
"Okay," she said.

Josie admits she was in a state of shock at
the time. "You don't know what to feel," she said.

"You don't know what to expect. My husband could be dying in the same second I am talking to this man. But he gave me a sense of calm. It's hard to describe it, but when you are in the hospital and somebody like Jerry comes along, it's like okay, I can breathe. It's okay, it will be okay, and that's basically what I took out of my first meeting with Jerry."

Josie then took Jerry up to Keli's room in the ICU.

"Is it okay if we shut off the lights, and close the curtains?" Jerry asked.

"Sure," Josie said, as she did as she was asked. "Is there anything else I can do?"

"No," Jerry said

Jerry was shocked when he first saw Keli lying there on his bed in the hospital ICU. What he saw was a man with tubes coming out of him, with a still bloody and severely swollen face. All kinds of monitors were running, still illuminated in the darkened room. Keli was just lying there motionless. It was sad, very sad, and Jerry knew right away that Keli was hurt critically. One side of his head was swelled up like a balloon. So Jerry took a look and started working on him right away.

"I calmed myself and focused just as I do every time I begin working with someone," Jerry said. "I knew I shouldn't touch Keli. The injuries were so fresh and open there was no way I was going to actually place my hands on his head.

Instead, I generated a field and extended it from my hands."

Jerry said, "As I moved through his head I saw several places beneath the skull that were still seeping blood. I progressed the scene forward in time and saw this would at worst cause death, and at the very least cause brain damage. I also saw this was not Keli's path. Within a few minutes I had recreated the integrity of those areas and saw the seeping had stopped. A few minutes more and I had caused the body to begin washing away the blood that remained there. I knew this area would be fine within a short time. There was extensive damage to Keli's face, and this is where I placed my attention next."

Jerry explained that when he sees broken bones, it looks as if the field itself has been shattered. "The body desperately attempts to resolve the deformity by throwing massive energetic forces to the injured area. Because the trauma is so great the body also has to deal with pain and tissue damage. The restoration process is slowed due to the need of the body to attend each area in turn, modifying each injured area and in turn slightly restoring one section at a time. To the observer it looks like a slow process to heal the bone. The reason is that the body can only do so much at any given time to restore itself. Because Keli's injuries were so vast, the body was overwhelmed."

In Keli's instance, Jerry said, only marginal energy was present. "Keli's body was more involved trying to keep him alive. So, I took over and directed the events, adding energy to Keli's template. Within a few minutes I saw the field restructuring itself back into its proper shape and strength."

Tony Arnold, who accompanied Jerry and Josie up to the room, said he'd never seen anyone in such bad shape. Even though Jerry had worked on Tony's shoulder so he could throw a baseball again without any pain, Tony didn't think there was any possibility Jerry could help this man – he was too severely beaten.

Josie said it looked like both Jerry and Tony were praying for her husband. "He was just kind of silent at first," she said. "He was just kind of praying." Jerry and Tony were on one side, while Josie watched from the foot of her husband's bed. "After he said his prayer in silence, he took Keli's hands and he put his hands on various parts of Keli's body. He just kind of moved his hands," Josie said. "In certain places he would hold his hands still in that area. It was almost like a person working, trying to do something, something spiritual."

When Jerry moved his hands behind Keli's shoulder, he asked Josie if he had been hurt there. Josie said yes, he had a deep cut behind his shoulder.

Jerry described the healing as he does many others. "I took a look inside and started working on him," Jerry said. "I went inside and fixed the bleeding of his brain and reversed all that. Then I went inside to his organs and started working on those." Jerry said he also tried to fix the man's wounded spirit. "I also tried to soothe the trauma his spirit had endured."

"During the healing session with Keli I felt drawn deep into a vision," Jerry said. "I followed where the vision took me and found myself standing upon a vast green field. There, just ahead of me, I saw Keli lying on his back on the grass. His eyes were closed, as if he were sleeping. I kneeled down and ran my hand across Keli's forehead and shook his shoulder. As his eyes opened, I stood up and told him he needed to wake up and follow me. I told him 'You can't stay here. You're going the wrong way.' Keli just looked up at me and nodded, and the vision was finished as suddenly as it had started."

Like many other people who experience a healing with Jerry, Josie noticed the hospital room seemed to warm up while Jerry was working on her husband. "It seemed warm and very quiet at the same time," Josie said, "which is kind of strange because Keli had all these machines hooked up to him in the ICU, all these beeps, and all these sounds. But when Jerry did his thing, everything just kind of stilled and calmed. It was the weirdest sense of warmth and then quietness...and you just don't really picture anything. Everything else seems blocked out, all you feel is this warm sensation and you are very at ease. You can almost feel him moving his hand. You can feel it with him."

After Jerry finished, they walked outside, and Jerry asked about Keli's back.

Josie said, "Yes. He's always had problems with his lower back because he's always lifting heavy construction materials."

Jerry told her he had managed to fix most things, but that Keli would still have some problems with his back. Then he told her, "Don't worry about it. Your husband is going to be fine. Don't believe what the doctors are telling you. That's just their job. But I'm telling you your husband is going to be just fine."

Josie looked stunned, not comprehending what Jerry said.

He tried again. "He is going to be okay, Josie, really." Jerry said. "He will come out of his coma tomorrow. He's going to have one heck of a headache, but he is going to be okay. By tomorrow he will be awake and coherent." Jerry also told her there was nothing he could do right now about Keli's brain swelling, but that in a few days it would go away as well. He had worked on improving the fluid flow through her husband's brain. A large tube was draining blood and excess fluid from her husband's injured skull, and Jerry said he would make sure the brain drained properly so Keli's brain could heal. He also worked on Keli's eyes. But again he reassured her that Keli would be okay.

Tony Arnold looked back at where Keli's room was and couldn't believe his friend was telling Josie that. It still looked to him like Keli could die any moment.

But the delayed effect on Josie was profound. "I was extremely ecstatic," she said later. "You can't really explain it. You're not only in a state of shock, but I'm also hoping that my husband will be okay. All these things are going through your mind, and this man just told me my husband was going to be okay. I was just so relieved." A huge sense of relief swept over Josie. "That's wonderful, that's what I needed to hear. I knew right after Jerry said that that my husband was going to be fine. Whatever the doctors told me, he was going to be fine."

Jerry also told Josie about his vision of Keli lying in a field of green grass. "I told Josie about this to let her know Keli was resting and present. I believe there are times the spirit leaves the body when the situation is critical. I wanted Josie to know Keli was still present." Jerry said.

Keli came out of his coma the next day.

Still on a respirator for a few more days, he had to wait before he could communicate with his wife, which he did mostly by pointing at things. The first thing he wanted to do was go home. But he had more healing to do.

When he could finally speak, he told Josie about a dream he had. "He woke up," Josie said. "And he told me about his dream. He said this really tall man was walking up to him. He was trying to wake him up. But Keli was walking away, walking away. He said this really tall man kept shaking him on his shoulder, like wake up, what are you doing? You are going the wrong way. That's when Keli woke up." At this point, Josie hadn't told her husband about Jerry yet. But she knew immediately who Keli was dreaming about. Once he said "really tall man," she knew it had to be Jerry. "When he said that, it was like, oh my gosh!" Josie said. "Then I told him all about Jerry." This was apparently the "healing of a wounded soul" and the vision Jerry had mentioned to her.

A year after the attack, Keli and Josie still live in their south Phoenix home. The big barrel-chested Tongan still does not work regularly, and still has problems with one of his eyes. But the damaged eye is the only sign of the brutal attack that almost killed him. He walks and speaks normally, and he credits Jerry. "He saved my life," Keli said.

Remembering the day he regained consciousness in the hospital, Keli said, "When I woke up, Josie told me about everything that had happened. How the doctors wanted to pull the plug. Then she told me about Jerry. Right away I wanted to call him; I wanted to meet him."

A week or so after the attack, Keli had been transferred to the hospital's physical therapy ward, and Jerry came for a visit. Keli was excited to finally meet him. "I was already excited," Keli said. "Because I knew I was going to go home soon. So the next day, I told my wife I wanted to see Jerry. So she called him, and he said he would come around five or six o'clock the next day. When he walked in the door, I thought this is one big guy. And he came in and gave me a hug and asked how I was doing. I said okay. I told him thank you for coming and seeing me when I was in ICU. He said he prayed for me."

Keli also thought he felt the spirits of other people in the room when Jerry came to visit, people who were interested in Keli's recovery.

During his second visit, Jerry did some follow-up work. As in many of the more complex cases Jerry works on, it sometimes requires an extra visit or two to help keep his client's body on the path to recovery. "He worked on me again, and I felt stronger," Keli remembered. "When he touched me, I felt heat. His hands were very warm. And I felt like singing when he touched me. And we prayed some more for my left eye."

It was hard for Keli to talk then; he still had a tube in his throat to help him breathe. "I wanted to ask him why God saved my life," Keli said.

The day after Jerry's second visit, Keli got out of bed and walked up to his nurse. He said, "Look, I'm well enough to go home now."

The nurse was shocked. In fact, ever since Jerry's first visit, doctors and nurses were unable to explain Keli's recovery. "They don't have any explanation for it. They never have," Josie said. "They thought if he did survive that he was going to be brain damaged. They were shocked at his progress." Josie likes to joke that her husband is just as crazy as he ever was – thankfully.

Later that same day, Keli pointed to a piano the hospital kept for patients in the physical therapy waiting area. He wanted Josie to play something. Keli had often sung at his church, but hadn't been able to since the accident. "I wanted her to play the piano in the waiting room," Keli told me later. "I wanted to sing."

As Josie began to play, Keli, remarkably, began to sing. The nurses nearby were amazed. His doctor said he's never heard of anyone being able to sing after a tracheotomy. But there he was, singing away with his wife playing the piano.

Keli was singing "Nearer the Cross" in his native Tongan. "I don't know the words in English," Keli said. "She played, and I sang. Then she said she was tired, and I said okay, I'll play. So I played the piano, and I sang. I didn't know anyone was standing behind me, but my doctor was there. He told me I was doing a great job."

Both Josie and Keli's doctor stood there and watched in amazement. "His doctor told me that it was the first time he's ever seen anyone with a tracheotomy actually try to sing," Josie said. "He said they usually can't even talk… he was like, wow!"

Jerry met the couple sometime later, and told them he knew they were trying to have a baby. "We don't have any kids yet, but he kind of looked into the future and he said don't worry about it, you'll get there, don't worry about it," Josie said. "He said I can see you guys on an island, and I can see you pregnant, so don't worry about it."

About a year later, Josie gave birth – on the island of Tonga with Keli at her side.

Keli and Jose met up with Jerry one more time, at an open house Jerry held. "He came over with his wife and just sat there quietly while all this activity and bustle was going on," Jerry said. "I was meeting and greeting and talking, and I saw him sitting there. Finally I got freed up and went over and knelt down in front of him. I said, 'How are you? It's good to see you.' He said, 'I just came by. I just wanted to see your place and to see you and say hello, and thank you for saving my life.' For a guy who looks as big as a grizzly bear, just a big guy like a football player, it was an amazing moment. He said, 'I just wanted to thank you for saving my life.'" Jerry said the big Tongan had a little tear in his eye. "I said, 'Hey, what are friends for?'"

The entire episode was a humbling one for Jerry. "I see miracles a lot. I see the effects they have on people's lives. But to see someone who is supposed to be dead sitting there with someone who loves them, that they have this love, it was amazing. They are looking at their future life together, the happiness, all the joy, all the things that come with life. To know that he's going to have that future just touches me very deeply in my heart to the point where I could get a big tear in my eye. It's such a good thing to help someone like that, to have a chance to do one more good thing."

It was on June 2nd, 1990, that Phoenix radio disc jockey Dennis McBroom hurt his back. He was coming down a tower at the Mesa Amphitheater, carrying two tool boxes. Work lights were supposed to be switched on, but for some reason the system was out. Climbing down in the dark, Dennis took a wrong step, and the result was a wrecked spine. He had two reconstructive surgeries that left him more than an inch shorter than he had been. "While they gave me my lungs, my legs, my love life by what they did, they left me in pain," Dennis said years later. "I was basically going to be on pain management the rest of my life, which meant I was on a variety of drugs of varying strengths from the second surgery on. It wasn't a fun way to live, but manageable up to a point. It was very, very painful."

Dennis grew up in Phoenix. He wasn't a very healthy or strong boy. He had asthma, and he was one of those kids always carrying around an inhaler, constantly puffing on it every time he started to wheeze. "I grew up the asthmatic little kid, the guy you see sitting on the sideline with an inhaler when you are playing football. I was also allergic to everything, including my mother's milk," Dennis said. "It took two weeks for the doctors to figure out what I could eat."

But when Dennis turned twelve, his parents changed doctors. And Dennis met Mr. Arizona, who was a body building champion, but also asthmatic. "He was built to beat the band," according to Dennis. "And he lifted weights until it made his asthma better. Six weeks later I had a weightlifting set, and I've never stopped." Dennis said weightlifting kept him alive through a lot of things. "I broke my back that day, and got up and walked away."

After his spinal surgery, Dennis suffered another setback. He had a heart attack. "In a five year period I went through two major spinal surgeries…and then three years ago, heart surgery. Because I pumped iron since I was twelve-years-old, basically I had a strong heart, and had built up a collateral blood supply. So I had enough to survive so they could do a double bypass. I had two arteries that were completely blocked."

After suffering spinal pain for so many years, a friend recommended Dennis go see Jerry Wills. But at first, Dennis resisted. "I went off on a trip, and came back from that trip a few weeks later in terrible pain. My friend picked me up from the airport and told me we are going to see Jerry…it's time."

When Dennis was introduced to Jerry, it seemed like he had known him a long time. The same was true for Jerry, who had recognized Dennis's name from CB radio broadcasts he used to hear as a teen growing up in Kentucky. "It turned out that people would send audio cassettes of my old shows on KDKB," explained Dennis, who hosted alternative rock broadcasts on the then groundbreaking Phoenix radio station. "They would send them to these guys down south, and they would broadcast them over CB radio. They would rebroadcast KDKB shows, and that's how Jerry knew me."

Both Dennis and Jerry shared a passion for music. "That first time we talked music, we talked radio, we talked what it was like then here in Phoenix, and what it was like for Jerry back in Kentucky. It was like two old hippies getting together."

The two men formed an immediate friendship. "How can you not get along with that man?" Dennis asked. "You walk in, and you know, before you've said a word you know this is a nice guy, a good man. It's what he emanates. This man is energy."

After their chat, Jerry took a look at Dennis's back. "I'm a diabetic, so he looked at my endocrine system, too. He said the damage to my back was too far in the past to do anything more than what I was already doing…which was diet and exercise. But then he shut the pain off. And I mean shut it off." For the first time in more than fourteen years, Dennis felt no pain in his back.

"It was pain that was altering my life," Dennis explained. "It was the pain that was making me sick; it was the pain that was making me less than a whole person. And he shut that off. When we came out of the treatment room, it was obvious. He could feel the pain I had experienced. You could see it had taken a toll on him. The first thing he said to me was, 'You walk around with this every day?' I said yes. He said, 'You don't have to do that anymore.' We talked for a few more minutes. He had some water, and then he was fine." Dennis asked how he did it – how he got rid of the pain. Jerry told him he tries to put the pain on himself, and then gives it to God. "To me," Dennis says, "growing up and going to church as a kid, you were taught you had certain gifts and talents and they were up to you to use and develop. But they were gifts from God. Jerry's got one great gift. Well, he's got more than one. But that one in particular, that he can take that and let it go."

Later that same week, Dennis returned the pain patches, the Soma and other drugs that he was taking to his doctor to give to other patients. "I didn't need them anymore," he said.

It's been several more years now since Jerry treated Dennis, and he remains pain free. In fact, Dennis hasn't worried about it since that first night after he was treated. "After our session, I went home and went to bed, hoping I would still be pain free the next day. That next morning I got up, just rolled out of bed, stood up straight and I was fine-- none of this hanging onto my bed trying to get my back to straighten out, trying to pull the spasms out, which was what I had done every morning. I was just getting out of bed and starting my day moving around pain free. I have been ever since."

Dennis, who still carries a body-builder's physique, resumed his strenuous workouts in the gym. "I started doing stuff in the gym I haven't been able to do in years," Dennis said. "Plus I'm much nicer to live with, according to my wife, and I have to agree with her because I'm happier with me."

Dennis also ended up taking a healing class from Jerry (More on Jerry's classes later) and took to it quickly himself. In fact, Dennis had been trained in massage and acupuncture even before his injury. "I've got twelve-hundred school hours and a little over ten-thousand practical hours in massage. I started acupuncture in 1992, so I don't have as many hours in that, but I've done a lot of it," he said.

Dennis started doing massage when he was ten-years-old, when his doctor said he could help his mother with her migraines. "It was the first time I figured out you can help people with your hands," he said. "And a while later, I figured out there is an energy involved there, and it's easy to help other people."

Dennis remains close to Jerry; the two often share their experiences. Dennis always remains impressed with what Jerry can do. "Jerry is on one hand a very big man, and on another hand a very gentle man," Dennis said. "He has an incredible gift and he uses it to help people. The bottom line: anyone who needs to know Jerry Wills should know that the guy is a big, tall, gentle giant. And he can make you better. Just trust him and let him do it, because he is the real deal."

Julie is an attractive young woman who lived and worked in Phoenix. She also owned a horse she kept in a stable in nearby Gilbert, Arizona. She learned about Jerry Wills and suggested that her father, a North Dakota rancher, see Jerry for a number of physical ailments that were bothering him. So that's what Gene Fedorenko did when he was in Phoenix in August, 2006. Jerry worked on him at Jerry's home in Peoria, and afterwards Gene felt much better. Among other things, the pain in his legs and feet was gone.

After he told his daughter about the visit, Julie got another idea. Her horse was hurting. There was something wrong with his left front leg that the vet couldn't pinpoint, saying it might require very expensive surgery. Julie decided to see if Jerry could come out and see her horse.

Jerry agreed, and the next day headed out to where Julie's horse was kept, at a small horse stable near some rodeo grounds in Gilbert, Arizona, which is not far from Phoenix. There were two horses in the corral which was bordered by a white fence and a small mobile home. Julie met Jerry at the gate. She owned one of the horses, a beautiful five-year-old quarter horse named Cutie. She had a long, deep black mane and a black tail.

The other horse in the corral was another quarter horse, this one, a twenty-eight-year old who had seen better days. His coat was coarse and scratched. A long white stripe on his nose was partially hidden by the blue fly shield over his head. His name was Quasar.

Julie took Jerry up to Cutie so he could take a look. Quasar walked up, too, and nudged Jerry with his nose. "Strange," Julie said about Quasar. "He's one of those horses who has served man while he has not been served." Quasar's owner was the man who managed the corral. He was nowhere to be seen. "Quasar usually doesn't like strangers."

"Hold on a minute, big guy," Jerry told Quasar. "I'll get to you in a moment." Jerry wanted to treat Cutie first. After all, she was the reason Julie wanted him to be there.

Jerry examined Cutie's left front leg. "The problem is down here," Jerry said as he pointed to the left front leg and ankle area of the horse. Jerry held Cutie's leg in one hand while his other hand was pressed to his forehead. He then kneeled and put both hands on the lower front left leg. Jerry seemed to be concentrating – just like he does when treating human clients. But again, Quasar came over to nudge him.

"Come on, Quasar," Julie said as she tried to lead the horse away.

"You should have your dad keep both of them," Jerry said referring to Julie's horse and Quasar.

But Quasar wouldn't quit. "Listen," Jerry said, "give me a second, all right? I have to do this." Jerry then turned his attention back to Cutie.

At about that point, Julie's father Gene arrived, and joined his daughter as Jerry worked on Cutie.

After a few moments, Jerry told Julie to go ahead and let Cutie test the ankle. She took the lead from Jerry, walked Cutie to the center of the corral and then waved her hands in the air. The horse immediately bolted to the other side of the corral. Julie thought Cutie seemed to still favor her left leg a little bit. Jerry saw the same thing and went back to work on her.

After Jerry held the horse's ankle for another minute or two, Julie again coaxed the horse to a gallop inside the corral. Cutie didn't seem to favor the ankle as much. Jerry said it would take the horse some time to trust it, because some pain was still there. But she should be fine. "Get another x-ray in about a week," Jerry told her. "By then it should be healed."

Then Jerry said there was something else bothering Cutie, and Quasar, too. With an odd look on his face, Jerry scanned the corral and the nearby rodeo grounds with his eyes as if he were looking for something. "It's something about this place they don't like. They're telling me something about the ground, but I don't know what."

Remember Jerry's days on the farm growing up in Kentucky? He said he could communicate with animals by sharing visual images telepathically. Now he was getting an image from both horses that something was wrong with the corral.

"This corral and the rodeo grounds are built on an old landfill," Julie said.

"Oh, that must be it," Jerry said. "They don't like it here. Too bad you can't take them both away from here."

Now, finally, it was Quasar's turn. "Let's see what's bothering you," Jerry said as he walked up to the older quarter horse, and stroked him with both hands.

After just a few seconds, Jerry said, "There's something wrong with his shoulder." As the horse stood perfectly still, Jerry put one hand on the horse's front left shoulder, and moved the other to the horse's leg. As the two of them watched, Jerry told the horse, "Take a deep breath."

It wasn't what everyone saw next but what they heard that shocked them – a strange deep sound, like the rush of air through something large. They realized as they watched the horse's chest cavity expand, that the horse was taking a deep breath! They could hear the air rushing into his lungs, and they could see the horse's nostrils flare, and they saw his chest expand. He was taking a deep breath! This twenty-eight-year old horse Jerry had never even seen before had just taken a deep breath after Jerry asked it to. It was stunning. Then the horse exhaled, and his heavy breath even kicked up some of the loose dirt in front of him.

"Now, lift this leg," Jerry said. Quasar's left front hoof came off the ground. The horse held it there for a moment.

"Okay," Jerry said, and the horse put his hoof back on the ground.

"One more time, lift this leg," Jerry asked.

Again the horse raised his leg one more time.

"That should help you," Jerry said as he patted the horse. Quasar then walked back to his stall, seemingly satisfied with the attention he had finally gotten from Jerry.

When he was later asked about the verbal directions to Quasar, Jerry said it helped that Quasar understood English. "That's true of most older horses," Jerry said. "They are very smart. With Cutie I had to communicate visually, by creating certain images. Most animals communicate that way. But with Quasar, he understood everything I was saying. Makes it easier that way."

As he was about to leave, Jerry asked Julie's father Gene how he was feeling since his session the day before. Gene said he was much better, but he still had a little pain in his back and in the heel of one foot when he woke up. Jerry said, "Let's take a look." He worked on Gene's back and foot for a moment. Gene said that both felt better.

As they parted ways, Gene invited Jerry to visit him sometime at his ranch in North Dakota. Jerry said he would like that.

Later Jerry would say it was sometimes refreshing to work on animals. But he was still worried that both horses lived on what was once a landfill, and that it scared them. "Who knows what is in that landfill? Whatever it is, those horses really don't like it."

Jerry also wished he could have taken Quasar home with him. "That was one very cool, very intelligent horse," Jerry said. "I really hope he will be okay."

Jerry's Birth Certificate – for September 11, 1953
Note the place of birth: Ft. Knox, Kentucky

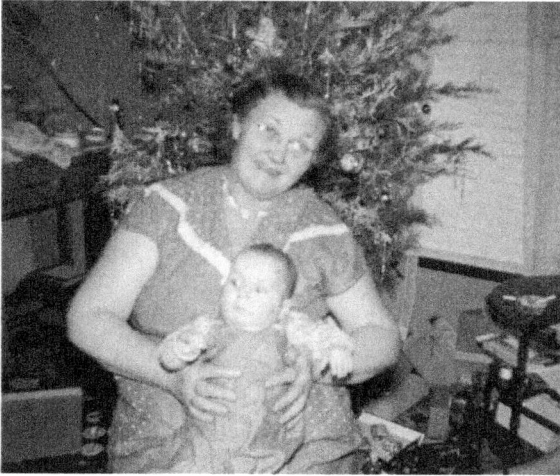

Jerry Wills with his grandmother, December 25, 1953 at home in Kentucky

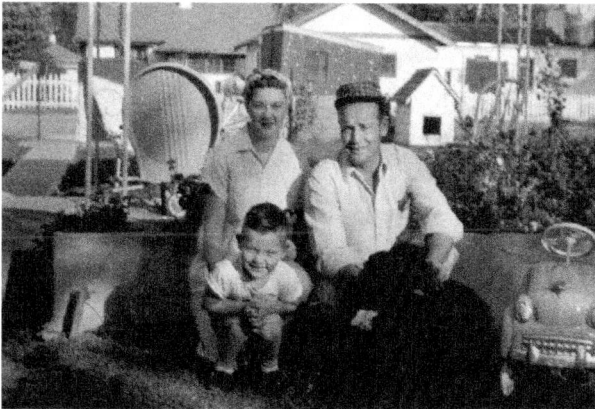

Jerry, Mother and Ace in front yard of Denver home

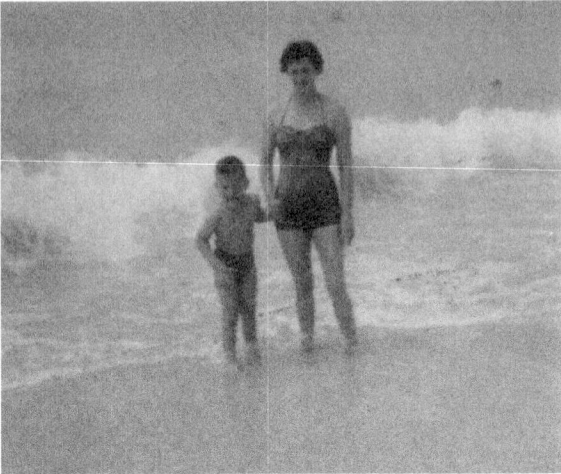

Jerry and Mom on Beach in Florida

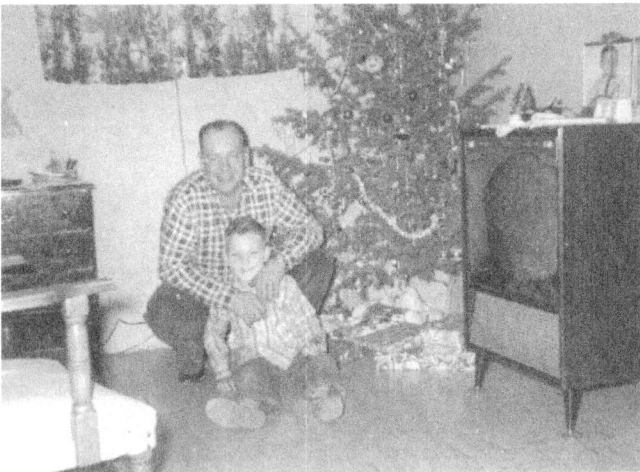

Jerry and father, Ace at home in Colorado

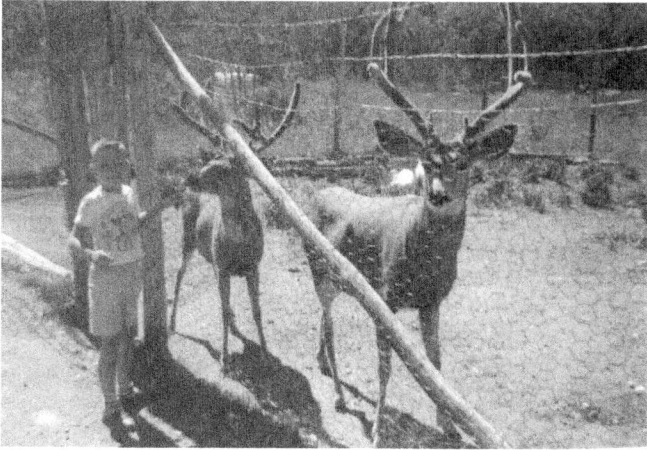

Jerry with deer at petting zoo near Denver

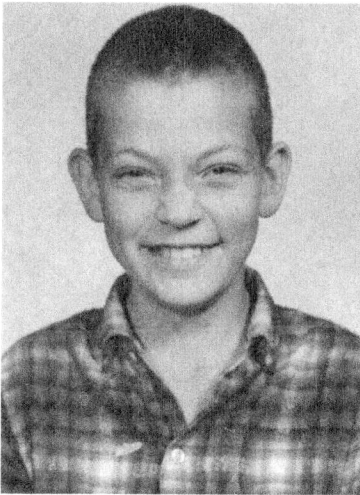

Jerry Wills School photo in 1963

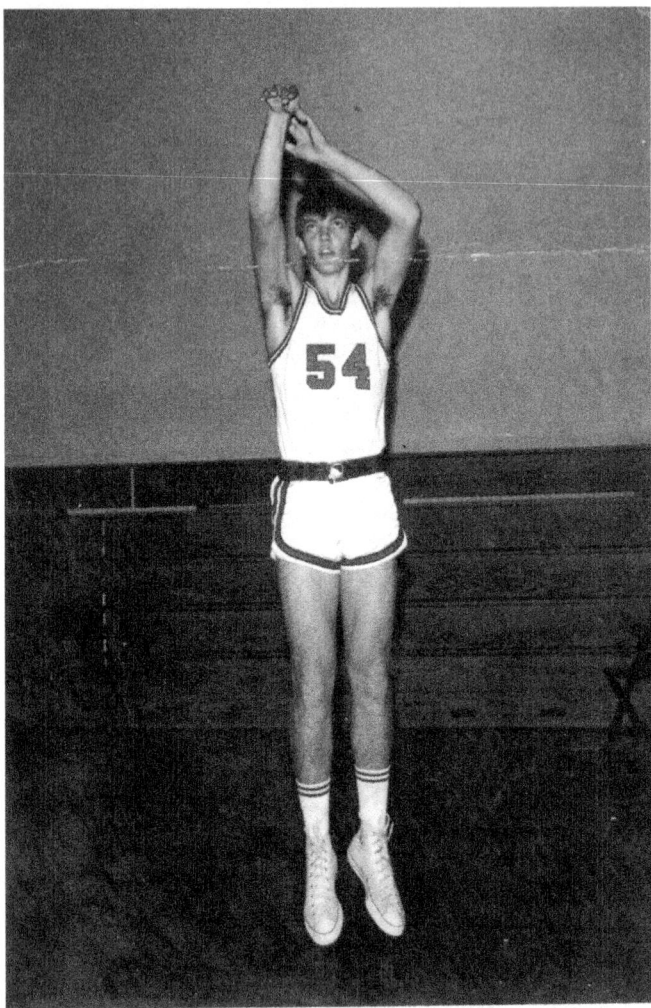

Jerry played center for the East Hardin High School
Rebels in Glendale, Kentucky

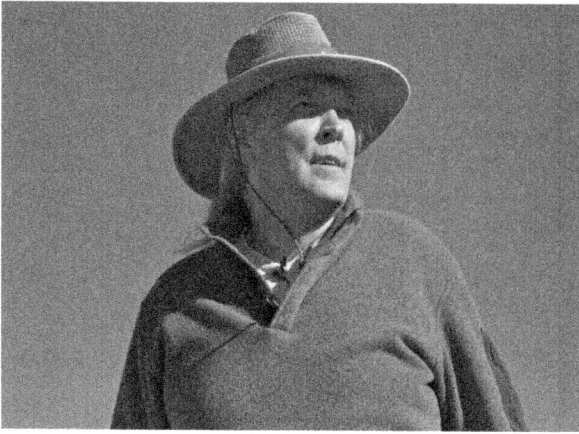

Jerry during 2008 expedition to look for lost city in the Andes Mountains of Peru

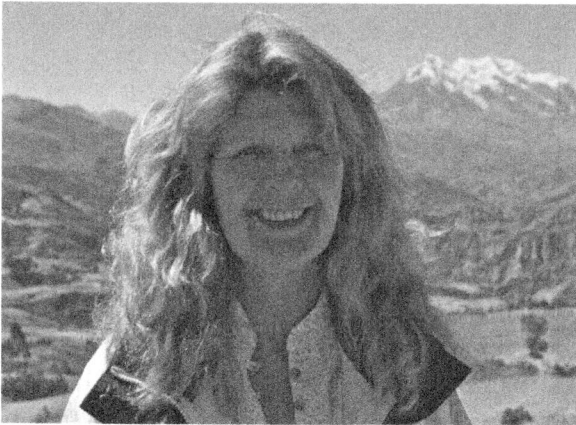

Kathy Wills during 2008 Bolivian expedition of the astrological alignment of Teohuanaco

Chapter Nine
Peruvian Expeditions

The South American nation of Peru is probably best known for its preserved archeological sites of the ancient Incan Empire. The ruins at Machu Picchu are visited by thousands of people every year. So are the mysterious Nazca lines, huge petroglyphs drawn in the desert that can only be seen in their entirety from the air.

Peru is the twelfth largest country in the world and is nearly twice the size of Texas. Moist, tropical jungles of the Amazon rainforest dominate eastern Peru. Lake Titicaca, the highest navigable lake in the world, lies along Peru's border with Bolivia. Southeastern Peru is made up mostly of a dry basin along the slopes of the Andes. And along the border with Chile lies the Atacama Desert – one of the driest places on Earth.

Lima is the capital city now, but Cuzco was the original Incan capital city, and center of an empire that thrived from 1438 until the Spanish arrived. The Incans worshiped Inti, the sun god. Medicine men, called shamen, were revered for their healing powers and wise counsel.

But it all unraveled when Spanish explorer Francisco Pizarro began his expedition to Peru in 1530. Most of his 2,000 soldiers turned back to Panama shortly after the expedition began. But with only thirteen men, Pizarro managed to capture the Incan Emperor who was weakened by civil war, and the Empire quickly fell.

After a predictable series of wars and military dictatorships that were so common in South America for centuries, Peru eventually became a republic and accepted its first constitution in 1979. It survived its first major challenge in 1980 when it put down a rebellion against the government by the Shining Path, a breakaway faction of the communist party in Peru, and remains fairly stable to this day.

But little of the ancient Incan Empire and its people remain.

As the Spanish conquered the lands that eventually became the nation of Peru, Catholic priests often followed the Conquistadors on their missions. They were an integral part of the destruction of indigenous peoples. They denounced every shaman they came across as a "devil worshiper" and often had him killed on the spot. It was a practice that continued for centuries. As late as the 1970's, historic petroglyphs were being defaced by missionaries in the Amazon.

Meanwhile, a young Jerry Wills growing up in Kentucky always had a fascination with far away places, though he didn't know why. As long as he can remember, he'd had a passion for lost cities and ancient mysteries. For Jerry, it was an unspoken, intangible type of thing. He didn't know where it was. Jerry imagined it must have been some sort of lost island or something like it. It was just a fantasy thing, but it was so real to Jerry, he thought he should know it. But at such a young age, he couldn't piece it together.

Then Jerry heard about a book called <u>Chariots of the Gods</u>. "It wasn't until I read Eric von Daniken's book that everything fell into place for me," Jerry remembered.

Jerry started reading everything he could about Peru. "I later read books by David Hatcher Childress. Many of his books dealt with little known facts he picked up and his adventures as he traveled through South America. There were just so many mysteries about South America. At times it was like reading about another planet. It just sounded so interesting."

Jerry was also a big science fiction fan. "I liked 'Star Trek.' I liked 'Lost in Space,' anything science fiction, whether it be a movie or television program," he said. "But here was something that's not science fiction. It talked about science fiction-sounding events, but it's real. So I knew I had to get there someday, somehow."

Jerry also read books about shamanism and found the subject fascinating. "I had never done anything approaching what they had done, but I thought it was interesting, and I wondered about the potentials. It felt like there was something there I should know."

Before he knew it, Jerry had an offer to go to Peru, to be a guest host for a tourist excursion still in the planning stages. "I just made friends with this guy," Jerry explained. "He didn't have anyone going to Peru. He was just trying to put together a tour, and no one was signing up. I told him I'd been all over the world doing lectures, and I offered up my mailing list. It was huge."

Jerry asked the man how many he needed to make the trip work.

He said, "Ten."

Jerry said, "Well, I got twenty." Jerry didn't make any money, but he got a free trip to Peru.

Jerry's first trip to Peru guiding his own group was in 1990, and he started taking tourists there twice a year. Along the way he met James Redfield, author of The Celestine Prophecy – a novel about ancient scrolls discovered in Peru. These scrolls included nine insights about the spiritual evolution of man that would become part of man's development as the new millennium approached. Jerry found the concepts fascinating. "It (the book) was good for spiritual connectivity and developing further," Jerry said. "The Celestine Prophecy was about personal evolution. It had a lot of really good lessons in it, so the tours I offered to Peru were based on The Celestine Prophecy. That meant they were experiential tours, a trip where you go to meet shamen, have experiences, and encounter moments of awakening."

During this time, Jerry was still married to his third wife. Sometimes his wife went on the trips with Jerry; sometimes she didn't. "Sometimes she did not go because there were too few passengers. But sometimes we needed to conserve the money because she had to pay just like any passenger would pay; so did I," Jerry said. "These trips were supplementing our income because I was still at work with electronics repair, and there wasn't much money in repairs as we progressed into the 1990's. Technology was changing in such a way that it was becoming cheaper to buy a new VCR or TV than to fix one that was broken."

Compared to what he had read, Jerry hadn't experienced anything special on his trips to Peru, which was disappointing. Until the one he took in 1997. "Everything was pretty much the same," Jerry said. "The jungle was interesting. Cuzco was interesting. Then we took the train and went to Machu Picchu. We got there in the afternoon. The vivid blue sky was filled with puffy cotton ball kinds of clouds."

Then they noticed several people were looking and pointing toward the sky. Something shiny was moving through the clouds toward them. "We were in the middle of Machu Picchu," Jerry explained. "There were several of us standing there watching as this shiny object moved through the clouds overhead. Within a minute or so it came closer and closer until it looked to be the size of a dinner plate. We all look at each other and exclaim, 'It's a flying saucer!'"

Jerry said it passed right over the group. "It was as shiny as a shiny nickel would be or a polished hub cap. Within moments it had moved over us, landing right on the saddle back of the nearby mountain. It sat there for the longest time."

The people gathered in that small group saw it. "Everyone was excited. They were just blown away," Jerry remembered. "News of our sighting spread quickly through our group of twenty-four, and everyone wanted to hike over to where the object landed. Of course, I'm the guy leading the tour. I'm supposed to know how to get over there. Well, I know how, and I knew it would take the better part of a day to get there." Jerry explained it would be difficult to hike to where the object was, and it was already two o'clock in the afternoon.

They decided against hiking. Instead a few people tried to take pictures of the object, but some low clouds rolled in, and their "flying saucer" was obscured along with the mountain where it had landed. The last thing seen were two or three figures moving around the craft. Finally, the group continued its tour of Machu Picchu without further diversion.

But that night, the group returned to Machu Picchu for a ceremony with a local shaman, C'ucho. Jerry said it was part of the normal routine. "This was one aspect of our trips I so thoroughly enjoyed. I have always enjoyed going up to Machu Picchu at night. It was just amazing with all the white granite glowing in the dark from the moonlight, and to see all the stars of the southern hemisphere."

As part of the ceremony, they placed two candles on the Temple of Pacha Mama, which Jerry said, "is a big stone, a temple to the feminine energy of the Andes."

Then with little warning, a thick fog bank moved in. Jerry remembered that, "It was so thick, you could cut it with a knife. It was astonishing. People were lying on the ground and being in this fog. You couldn't see anything, just the outlines of the ruins in the light from two candles."

As they watched, two llamas came into view. "They started dancing and playing; it was the strangest thing I've ever seen up there. The llamas were jumping up and down right next to our group. Their movement created these really long, dark, bizarre shadows. Meanwhile, the shaman is playing his flute and he's chanting and singing. The night was very magical."

By 1:30 in the morning, Jerry led the tour group back to a waiting bus which returned them to Aguas Calientes. It was a forty-five minute drive back down to Aguas Calientes, and a twenty minute walk to the gate at the Pueblo Hotel where they stayed. "Then you climb up all these large stone stairs to get to the hotel," Jerry recalled. "You get your key at the front desk, and you climb up even more stone stairs and walkways winding through the gardens there. By the time you get to your room, you are huffing and puffing and sweating and just going, 'Oh my God, I'm glad I'm here.' You sit down, wipe your brow, and try to catch your breath."

Jerry made sure everyone got to their rooms before he could completely relax. "Their rooms, actually individual bungalows, were spread throughout the compound," Jerry said. "But they were all within shouting distance."

He splashed cold water on his face to wash the dust off, brushed his teeth, and climbed into bed. Jerry was finally settled in for the night.

There was a little bit of a chill in the air, so Jerry grabbed an extra blanket. Suddenly, Jerry heard his name being called. "Jerry! Jerry!"

Sitting up in bed, Jerry thought someone was calling for him. He didn't recognize the voice, but the name was very clear.

Jerry got out of bed, put his clothes back on, and went to the door to look outside. But there was no one there. Jerry walked around the outside of his bungalow to take a look, but he couldn't see anyone. After a few minutes, he went back in, got undressed, lit a cigarette, and climbed back into bed.

Jerry had some of his own pillows propped up behind him. "Pillows down there are like sleeping on shredded tires shoved into a gunny sack. That's what a pillow feels like, and it's not very good. Always take your own pillows," Jerry said.

He finished his cigarette, switched off the bedside lamp, and closed his eyes. Then he heard a strange sound, like cellophane being crinkled up. He opened his eyes. Standing before him, inside his room, were seven people, just standing there at the foot of his bed in a semicircle, staring down at him. To Jerry they looked very tall, like nine or ten feet tall, their heads just below the vaulted ceiling in Jerry's room. And they were just standing there staring at him.

Frightened badly, Jerry pulled the blanket over his head. A few moments later, when he looked again, they were still there. There were tiny beads of light moving around and on the sides of their bodies. It also looked as if they were lit from behind somehow. It was the damnedest thing Jerry had ever seen in his life. Overwhelmed by the scene before him, Jerry took a breath, and then passed out.

When Jerry came out of it, his guests were still there. He pulled the covers over his head again and tried to stop shaking, and to clear his mind.

"I knew we shouldn't have done it this way," said a man's voice. "We've frightened him."

"No," said a woman. "It's going to be all right." Then she started calling Jerry's name. "Jerry, it's going to be all right. Don't be afraid. We didn't mean to scare you. We're not here to hurt you. But we really need to speak with you. Please, don't be afraid of us."

Jerry, still under the covers, felt there was something very compelling about the way she spoke to him. Feeling reassured, Jerry felt that maybe it was okay.

To be safe, Jerry remained underneath the covers. His teeth clenched, his eyes squeezed tight, hands in a death grip on the sheet pulled over his head. Later, Jerry thought, "It must have been quite funny seeing a grown man doing that."

Jerry slowly pulled himself up over the sheet to see what was going on. He saw the people again, still standing there. But he still didn't say anything.

"We are here to deliver a message," one of them said.

After that, they discussed Jerry's life and told Jerry it was time to make a choice. "I don't remember all the details of what they said," Jerry said later. "It was just so mind-blowing. I do remember the general nature of it. They wanted me to know that it was time to make a choice. That the way my life was going could continue if I wished, or I could decide to do what I had come here to do. That if I made the decision to do what I was here to do, my life was going to change dramatically. And if I chose to fulfill my life's mission, the decision would require me to endure heartache and sweeping changes the like of which I had never experienced before. I remember telling them I could only choose to do that which I had come here to do regardless of the consequences. I simply could not waste the opportunity available to me to be of service no matter the cost."

Jerry didn't say much more than this. He just listened to what they had to say. They accepted his answer saying, "Please know this will not be easy. But the choice you have made will influence and enrich many lives. Know we are always ready to help you if called." A moment later, they were gone - vanished back into the night. They simply were no longer there. There wasn't any mist or residual twinkling of light that floated off through the window or anything like the movies. They just vanished in the blink of an eye.

Jerry thought to himself, what did I eat to make this happen? He was pretty shaken and exhausted. It had been a long day, and soon he drifted off to sleep.

The next day, Jerry's tour group was scheduled to see another shaman at a place Jerry called The Waterfall of Dreams. Jerry was late getting up, and after a quick breakfast, he headed out after his tour group. He rejoined them as the shaman began his ceremony.

Jerry noticed that there was someone else at the waterfall as well. This older fellow had spread out an old red cloth about three feet by three feet upon the ground and offered coca leaf readings for Jerry's group. Jerry knew this was typical. He had seen the locals do coca leaf readings, and it cost about five bucks. It was part of the magic that is Peru. Even if it's not entirely legitimate, Jerry was thinking those on the tour would still enjoy it.

Jerry watched the coca leaf reading for a few minutes. He was fascinated just watching and listening as the old man spoke Ketchua, the ancient language of the Inca. The old man also wore an old, weathered fedora hat that was faded and crumpled from the years.

Awhile later, C'ucho came up to Jerry with the old coca leaf reader in tow. He said the old man wanted to do a leaf reading for Jerry.

Jerry said, "No, that's okay. Just do the passengers; I'm leading this trip. His time should be spent with them."

"No, I want to for you," the old man said in his best broken English.

"That's okay, I'm not interested," Jerry repeated. Jerry thought he'd already had enough weird stuff happen in the last twenty-four hours. He didn't need anymore.

The old man looked disappointed as Jerry walked away.

As the tourists headed back, Jerry decided to stay behind a few more minutes and enjoy the waterfall by himself. After all, he had a lot to think about. The UFO sighting and the people he saw in his room the night before were something that he couldn't quite get a handle on. Then there was the mention of his life changing in dramatic and unpredictable ways. What could this mean? What was going to happen? Had it already started? Jerry felt troubled and tired.

The jungle was filled with glistening drops of water floating on the air currents as the sun started dropping behind the mountains. It was a beautiful and calming sight – especially after the tourists had left. After about a half hour or so, Jerry headed back.

He was walking by himself, thinking about what had happened the night before, and he was beginning to think that it wasn't real, that it couldn't possibly have happened. He must have been dreaming. It just can't be like that.

However, Jerry did consider carefully one thing his visitors said, that if he needed help from them, if he needed something, to just ask. So as Jerry walked along the railroad tracks that led back to town, he thought about asking for help. He wanted to know if his visitors were real or not. How would they answer? What if they reappeared again? Jerry wasn't sure he was ready for that.

The old railroad tracks were covered with black oil. The railroad ties reeked of it. As Jerry walked along he noticed one of his boots had come untied, and the laces were now a black oily mess. He bent down to tie his shoes, and right there at his feet was this perfectly square piece of alabaster. It was perfectly white. And it was instantly significant to Jerry because of something he had read about in a book titled <u>The Zen of Pooh</u>: that God is the un-carved block of stone. Jerry believed that as soon as you create an image of what God is, you've polarized God and therefore limited the true nature of God. In his mind that seemed pretty real. Jerry always liked that concept, that God was the un-carved block of stone.

And here before him was this stone. And it wasn't just another oily rock, but a beautiful, perfectly white piece of alabaster, right there at his feet. His shoes were untied, and covered with oil. It's the only reason Jerry bent over in the first place.

Jerry picked up the stone and took a closer look. There was not a bit of black oil or tar on it anywhere. It was perfect. And there wasn't anything else white anywhere around it. There was no alabaster to be found anywhere nearby.

Jerry took a few minutes to actually look for more alabaster in the surrounding area. Later, Jerry even asked the shaman about it. He was told there was nothing else like it there, maybe farther up into the mountains. The shaman said he only knew of a place four or five days away where you might find alabaster.

Then Jerry thought maybe he was trying to find something to give reason that the night before was real, and was stretching things a bit. Jerry put the rock in his pocket and forgot about it.

Later back in town, Jerry was having a Coke and just relaxing in C'ucho's office with his friend Edith, when C'ucho and the old coca leaf reader reappeared. Again, the old man said he wanted to read the leaves for Jerry.

"Okay," Jerry said, not wanting to disappoint the old man twice in one day. "I'll let you read leaves for me."

The old man flashed a mostly toothless grin and nodded in approval. He was clearly pleased and excited to begin.

Jerry's friend Edith and C'ucho pulled out a milk crate and put a square plywood board on top of it, turning it into a small table. The coca leaf reader then spread out his old red cloth like he had done for the tourists just a few hours before. Jerry sat on a narrow wooden bench against the wall of the narrow office. The makeshift tabletop was just below his knees.

The old man sat next to C'ucho, then took a bag off his back that he'd been carrying. It was full of coca leaves. He dumped them on the table.

The coca leaf reader then carefully went through his pile of leaves, picked out one leaf at a time and said a prayer as he held it delicately. Then he flicked it between his thumb and forefinger. It flew through the air and landed on his red hand-woven cloth. He did this over and over, about five or six times. The old coca leaf reader did this with so much finesse that the coca leaves lined up in a nice straight row. He was clearly a pro.

But then the coca leaf reader started shaking his head no, and said something to C'ucho who sat across the table from them, something Jerry couldn't understand.

With a concerned expression Edith seemed to ask something in Spanish to C'ucho, and as Jerry watched, they were now all shaking their heads.

Jerry wondered what was going on. "Hey, translate for me, will you?" he asked Edith.

"Wait, he needs to do this again because something isn't clear to him," she said.

Then the coca leaf reader picked up all the leaves, shuffled them up, and then did it all over again. He seemed even more concerned this time, and the three of them discussed the events even louder, still in Spanish.

Jerry couldn't take much more of this. He said, "Edith, what is going on?"

"I don't know," Edith said. "But I'm going to find out. Don't worry. It will be okay."

The three continued to converse in Spanish, and Jerry wished he knew the language better. He got more and more agitated as they continued their conversation.

"Jerry," Edith asked, "please, will you give him your hand?"

"My hand?" Jerry asked.

"Yes, give him your hand."

Jerry reached his hand across the table. The coca leaf reader took Jerry's hand in both of his, and pulled it close to his face. Tears suddenly streamed down his face and he said more things in his native Ketchua language.

Then the coca leaf reader looked over at C'ucho, and continued to plead in Ketchua, and started softly kissing Jerry's hand.

"What the hell is this all about?" Jerry whispered to Edith.

"I'll try to translate for you," Edith said. "He says he has waited all his life to meet you, or someone like you. You are fulfilling a prophecy that was told to him a very long time ago and has been given generation to generation. He was told that one day there would be angels who walked upon the Earth who have special gifts. And that these people would be there to help others who are sick or injured, to help them be well again. When they begin to find these angels, it is a sign that the end of the world is at hand and they needed to prepare themselves and their people for the times ahead. The angels from the stars who walk the Earth would be there to help insure the good people would survive and carry the world into the new age. These angels are really messengers from the stars I think, Jerry, although he isn't sure where they are from. He is only aware their presence is the fulfillment of this ancient prophecy."

Jerry looked over at the old man who continued to cry and kiss his hand. He couldn't believe this was happening.

Edith continued to translate. "He said you are one of these angels, and that he's waited all his life to meet you. He wants you to know that he respects who you are and would do anything to help you with why you are here."

"Wow," Jerry said, as he pulled back his hand. He had goose bumps all over, and Jerry was thinking, "Oh my God, this is too damn weird."

"Thank you very much," Jerry said, clearly shaken by what the coca leaf reader had said.

But he didn't want to stay. He had to go to the bathroom, so Jerry quickly got up and left the small room.

A few minutes later, however, he returned and sat down again. He was both shocked and curious. "What else does he see for me?" Jerry asked Edith.

"He says that you are married now to a woman that you are going to divorce within six months. And that you have a business working with electricity, but that this business is going to close within a year."

Jerry felt numb and said nothing. He just stared at the coca leaf reader who continued to speak in Ketchua and cry.

"He says there is another one," continued Edith. "He says there is another person who is supposed to be with you. She is the one you are going to be with. She has come to this world to add her strength to yours and to help you. She has golden colored hair. You are going to find her. You don't know who she is right now, but you are going to find her."

"Where in the world am I supposed to look for this person?" Jerry asked. "There are lots of women with golden hair. How would I know?"

Edith said, "You will know who this person is. She lives in the heart. The shaman says you will find her in the land of the heart."

232

Jerry wondered what that meant.

C'ucho pulled out a map of the United States, and said, "It is here, someplace."

Then the old man took a stick and pointed it right at the center of the United States.

Edith, continuing to translate, said, "He says, in the heart."

"Well, that's Nebraska and Missouri," Jerry said. "I'm not ever going to Nebraska. And not very likely Missouri either."

Edith listened to the old man, then said, "Well, maybe a little beneath the heart."

Jerry said, "Well, I'm not going there either. Besides, I'm married, and I'm happy, and everything is fine."

Edith said, "He says it's all going to change. Something has happened and it is already changing. The coca leaves tell him so."

Jerry was thinking this was nuts. "First I see things popping into my room giving me a message," Jerry said. "Then I find this white rock, and now I've got an old man reading coca leaves telling me my life is going to change. So I'm fighting against all this stuff internally. I just couldn't believe these surrealistic events were happening. I felt insecure and distressed. What if this were really true?"

It was finally enough for Jerry, so he got up and left the office. He met up with the rest of his tour group, had some pizza and beer with them, and tried to put it all behind him.

It was not over for Jerry, however. The next day he led his tour group to the Sacred Valley. After a short train ride they checked into a hotel next to an old monastery. They got there late in the day; it was about five-thirty in the afternoon. And it was just turning dark, with a slight chill in the air.

Jerry was helping the hotel staff to unload everyone's luggage off the bus, and was the last one to come into the hotel lobby. When he walked in, he noticed a woman behind the counter staring at him with a very intense look. She was looking right at him. She didn't say anything; as she checked each person in and proceeded to the next, she kept looking for and then staring at Jerry. He thought it was pretty odd, but not that unusual since Jerry is so tall…sometimes people liked to gawk.

Jerry finally got his key and went up to his room. He did his best to avoid anyone in the lobby, especially the woman who was staring at him.

The next morning, Jerry was having breakfast and told Edith about the woman he saw in the lobby the day before.

"This woman is an old friend of mine," Edith told Jerry. "I've known her a long time. Tell me, Jerry, have you ever been here before?"

"No," Jerry said.

"No? Really? Well, come with me." Edith then led Jerry to a yard outside the hotel. The woman was there waiting for them.

The woman greeted Jerry warmly and said something to him in Spanish.

Again, Edith translated. "She said, 'I'm happy you've come back. How have you been?'"

Jerry shook his head and said, "What do you mean? I've never been here before. I don't think we've ever met."

Edith, who remembered what the old coca leaf reader had said, replied, "I showed her your rock. Just answer her questions, please."

Jerry said, "Okay. Tell her I've been fine, but I don't remember that I've ever been here. So being happy that I came back doesn't make any sense to me."

Edith told the woman what Jerry said.

The woman replied, and again Edith translated. "She says that there was a rose colored triangle that appeared to her, a triangle of light that was hovering above the grass here in her back yard. Suddenly a shaft of light came up out of it, and then went back down again, and that you were standing there. She says that you have come to her many times to talk to her about very intense spiritual things, to ask her to always protect this land because it is spiritual."

"Ask her what I looked like," Jerry told Edith.

"She says you were wearing similar clothes to what you are wearing now."

Jerry knew he always wears the same kind of clothes when he is running a tour, so it's easy for the passengers to pick him out of a crowd, as if he weren't tall enough anyway.

"She wants to know why you don't remember it," Edith said.

"Tell her I don't know why," Jerry tried to explain. "I don't have an answer for that. I also don't know what is going on, but this has been a very strange trip."

Edith pulled Jerry aside. "Look," she said, "There are some very powerful forces at work here right now. I think you have to see another friend of mine, in Lima, and talk with her."

Jerry said, "Sure. When?"

"Now," said Edith. Jerry had known her for years, and knew she was someone he could trust, especially when it came to spiritual matters.

Edith made some quick plans and later that day she and Jerry left his guests with other guides who would finish the tour. That afternoon, both Jerry and Edith were on a plane to Lima.

After arriving, they took a taxi to see Edith's friend. A housekeeper answered the door, and they were invited in. Eventually, an older woman showed up to greet them. She said she was happy that Jerry was able to make it and asked if Edith would please translate since she didn't speak better than broken English.

It turned out that this woman was the personal advisor to President Fujimori of Peru. She was also a psychic and someone very trusted throughout South America.

Jerry ended up spending the next six and a half hours with her. She told him everything about the tall people he saw in his room, all the details. She told him everything, including what he didn't even tell Edith. She told him about the old man and the coca leaves and his predictions, and about the woman they had met in the Sacred Valley. He didn't tell her anything, but she knew everything. To Jerry it was unnerving.

"You are here for a reason," she told Jerry. "Because we are at the end of this age of the world. Another age, a golden age is dawning, and you are here to help people wake up so that they will be able to carry on in the next age. You are a healer," she continued. "You have made a decision. Now it is time for you to do what you are here to do."

She went on to tell Jerry that he had to stop any doubts about being a healer, and that his life was indeed about to dramatically change. It was going to change enormously. "The foundation you have built your life upon to this point is made of sand," she said. "It's an illusion. It's going to crumble, and it is going away. You are going to be left with nothing. You are going to have to recreate it again on the foundation of who you really are. If you don't, then you are going to be miserable the rest of your life. Soon you must go to the heart to find your answers and one who is waiting for you there. But don't wait too long. I can see she is impatient and might not wait for long."

Over and over again, Jerry was hearing the same message, one he had trouble hearing and accepting.

"Yes, but, I am happily married. My business is going well. And I see no changes on the horizon, none at all," he told the woman.

"You are wrong," she said. "And soon you will see..."

Within a few days Jerry was on his way back to Phoenix, considering, but mostly dismissing, all he had heard. The tour was finally over and all the strangeness was thousands of miles behind him. Yet, what if it were all true? It wasn't something Jerry wanted to consider. It remained unclear how three separate events, seemingly unlinked to each other, could contain the same information. The uneasiness created a relentlessly churning weight in his stomach.

As you will soon read, everything they had predicted for Jerry would come to pass.

"My marriage was over in six months," Jerry said later. "My business was over in a year. Once I returned to Phoenix I discovered I had a speaking engagement offered to me in Kansas City, and while I was there I met this woman with the golden hair. And that first meeting was another strange event. It was just the most bizarre set of circumstances you can imagine. It was like science fiction. Everything I had based my life on was fading away. Everything was changing."

But was it a self-fulfilling prophecy? Maybe.

"When my marriage was going to hell," Jerry said, "it was my fault. It wasn't anything she did. We had our issues, but what married couple doesn't? It wasn't like she did something wrong; she did nothing wrong. She was not at fault. It was just that this event happened, and I had to redefine myself somehow. She could not go there with me."

"Anyway," continued Jerry, "I was in a real state of emotional distress. I was just beside myself with sorrow and sadness and anxiety. I felt so lost because everything, everything was gone or fading away quickly. I was really sad about the way things were."

Jerry continued to travel the country on a lecture circuit and continued to organize trips to Peru. He spent a lot of time with his friends for support, and his work with Peruvian shamen continued during his trips. The prophecies of that trip came true – at least up to this point. As for the rest, well, Jerry said only time will tell.

Chapter Ten
Kathy

The first thing Jerry Wills did after graduating high school had nothing to do with becoming a healer. He discovered sex, fell in love, and got married. "It was pretty much a shotgun wedding," Jerry said. "She was fourteen, and I was eighteen. She wasn't pregnant, but her family was certain that it was necessary that she get married."

Jerry was married for six years before his first divorce. Three children resulted from that marriage, a daughter and two sons: Christy, Sean and Jerry.

Then Jerry met and later married a woman from Michigan. "We stayed together five years. That didn't work out either," he said. Together they had one child, Jonathan.

Jerry was living in Arizona after his second failed marriage. After being single almost a year he met his third wife. They were married about nine months later, and stayed that way for seventeen years. "When I met her she was the manager of a custom t-shirt shop. We started dating and just hit it off. We had differences of opinion when discussing the mysterious and metaphysical, but that didn't affect the relationship at that time," he said.

On one of his trips as a tour guide to Peru, Jerry had a profound incident involving special visitors who convinced him it was time to pursue life as a healer. Similar to his near death experience years before, it was another awakening. The visitors told Jerry it was necessary to make a life choice. It was either time to get on with what he was on Earth to do, or continue with his normal life as a business owner and an electronics repairman. He had to choose one or the other; he could no longer do both. Jerry says he came back to Phoenix with his head screwed on sideways.

Jerry said he shared everything with his third wife. "Towards the end she decided I must have been infected with a brain virus. During our marriage she felt embarrassed because I was interested in UFO's and the paranormal. I was also interested in doing more of the healing thing, exploring crystals and all that New Age stuff. She was embarrassed by the fact that I was really into that sort of thing. I was becoming less and less satisfied with my business and the direction I felt compelled to remain dedicated to."

According to Jerry, when he started going public with his lectures and writing for magazines, his third wife felt people would think he was strange and wouldn't want to be around him because he was so weird. Jerry did not care how others might judge his interests. He simply wanted to follow his inner guidance. He knew something powerful was stirring deep inside. Jerry wanted to know if he could help others through his ability to heal with a touch. He wanted to develop his skills further. She didn't think that was a good idea.

She said, "Now you're talking about touching people and healing them? Do you know how bizarre this sounds!" She had seen what Jerry could do, but she didn't want him to do it publicly.

"One thing led to another," Jerry said. "And we got a divorce."

Suddenly there was Kathy. They met while he was in Kansas City to drum up clients for his Peruvian tour business. "I was invited to the event to present a lecture about my experiences while traveling through Peru. My goal was to generate interest that others would sign up for future trips I'd be offering," Jerry said. "I also lectured about Shamanism. There were about eighty people who attended. When I went back to my table, Kathy and a group of her friends were there. She missed the lecture, so her friends brought her over to the table to introduce her. They said, 'Hey, this is the guy. This is really interesting stuff, and you should talk to him.' I took her hand, to greet her, and it was like someone suddenly threw a switch. There was a vacuum. Everything stopped, and there wasn't any sound. I felt an intense electric charge moving through my hand, and felt completely surprised by the event. It wasn't that I couldn't let go. It was that I didn't want to let go. Time stood still, there was no sound. It ended as abruptly as it had started once I let go of her hand. I noticed the golden hair and suddenly realized she was the one I had been told about in Peru!"

243

Kathy felt the same thing. "When we shook hands, it was just so weird," she said. "Because this energy just ran up my arm, and it was like nothing else existed. Time stopped. Then someone said his name, and the event ended." Kathy didn't say anything to her friends at first, nor did she say anything about it to Jerry. "I didn't say anything to him about that because I thought it was just such a strange thing. You don't usually tell anyone about that kind of experience until you have time to think it through," she said.

Kathy grew up on a farm in Nebraska, and lived in Lincoln for about twenty years. The granddaughter of Czech immigrants, Kathy's immediate family consisted of three older brothers and three younger sisters, her mother and father. After graduating high school she went to a community college and graduated with a cosmetology license.

When she met Jerry she was working for a major delivery service, but soon quit after seven years there. She found it a difficult environment for a woman employee. There was little opportunity for advancement. So she struck out on her own, starting a small courier service in Lincoln. She delivered anything and everything, including pizza, to make ends meet.

Kathy's first marriage ended in divorce after a year and a half. Her second marriage also ended in divorce, but this time after seven years. There were three children: Bryce, Jordan and Jena.

After her second divorce, Kathy and her friends got on the path of self-improvement and self-enlightenment. "We would go to intuitive arts festivals, psychic fairs, or gem and mineral shows," she said. "There were not not many places you could find information or events in the heartland. So, we took road trips to events being held in surrounding states."

As soon as Kathy and her friends discovered there was an intuitive arts festival in Kansas City, they knew they had to go. "That's where I met Jerry," she said.

"It wasn't my intention to meet anyone, nor was I looking," Kathy said. "With my work schedule and raising three children I had no time for romantic relationships. My friends were always looking for me but I wasn't interested, much to their disappointment. It takes a lot of emotional strength and time to nurture a romantic relationship. Besides, I had not had much luck finding men who were kind, honest or gentle. Instead, they were usually lazy or drank too much and some were even violent! Days before I left for Kansas City I had decided to stop looking. I swore off men," she said. "I'm not going to have anything to do with men for now. I was tired of the games. I made a decision to focus on me, my business and my kids."

Once in Kansas City, it was her friends who first saw Jerry. One friend was always trying to set Kathy up, and she thought Kathy would be very interested in Jerry because of their shared interest in Peru.

After their first dramatic meeting, Kathy and her friends went off to look at some of the artwork and visit the other booths lining the pavilion. But one of her friends continued to pester Kathy about Jerry. "Why don't you go over there and invite him to our hotel room to talk about Peru?"

Kathy resisted at first. But she eventually agreed and returned to the table Jerry had set up with brochures about his Peruvian expeditions. "One of my friends just got back from Peru," she told Jerry. "She has pictures and souvenirs, and wants to show them to you... and, ah... they want to invite you to hear about what you have experienced in Peru." Kathy babbled on, "You don't really have to go, but they want you come."

"Sure," Jerry said. "That sounds like fun. What time?"

"Ten o'clock," Kathy replied.

And at ten o'clock he was there. Kathy said they had a great time talking about Peru. Then Jerry and Kathy went down to the lobby, and they talked some more, until about two o'clock in the morning.

They met again the next day. "We hung out for awhile," Kathy said. "And he gave another lecture about Peru. Then we exchanged phone numbers. It was a friendship kind of thing."

Kathy knew nothing about Jerry's ability as an energy healer until the day she left Kansas City.

When Kathy was getting in her friend's Jeep, she grabbed the door handle and pinched her pinky finger in the door latch. She instantly had a nasty blood blister on her finger.

Jerry had taken a break from his booth to see them off and noticed what happened to Kathy's finger. He said, "Let me take a look at that." Then he took Kathy's hand.

She said, "Ouch, don't do that. It hurts. Stop it. What are you doing?"

Jerry then let go of her finger, and said, "The swelling will be down by the time you get home. Tomorrow you might not even notice it was ever hurt."

Kathy thought, yeah, right. She said, "Thank you, Jerry," and gave him a little kiss on the cheek as they left.

Two hours later they were nearly home. Kathy noticed the swelling on her finger was nearly gone. "I swear," she said, "the swelling was down within two hours, and it didn't hurt within fifteen minutes of him doing it. The next day, I couldn't even tell it was there."

Kathy wasn't sure what to think. She remembered, "I thought there was something strange about this guy. Jerry and the healing of my finger were mysterious, and I like mysterious things."

A few days later, she called Jerry. She said, "That's pretty wild what you did. How did you do that?"

Jerry said, "It was just energy. I directed it to change. Once I had done this, your body could easily absorb the blood, to then put it back in your system and repair the tissue. Everything is energy. Your body is energy. The molecules of solid matter are not moving as fast as other forms of energy. I affected the way your body handled the injury. Once restored, it allowed your body to go back the way it was."

For Kathy, it was hard to understand at first. She told her friends later that she didn't know what to think. The experience was very exciting and interesting. She wanted to know more.

Kathy had already experienced Reiki healing. "Reiki is something that helps you become familiar with directing energy by matching a symbol in your mind and directing energy the way the symbol flows," Kathy said. "But Jerry uses his consciousness without a symbol. That's a more ancient technique. It's the creative force inside he is working with. Working with energy the way Jerry does allows you tap into a part of yourself so many are trying to access."

Kathy and Jerry stayed in touch. "I met him again in June, and later in July he came to Nebraska. My friends and I had planned a trip to go tubing down the Niobrara River in north-central Nebraska. We invited Jerry, and he came along."

At the time, Jerry was going through his divorce. And Kathy wondered what she was doing. "I know how troubling emotionally it can be to go

248

through a divorce. It was really hard on me and I didn't want to go through this with him. I couldn't stand the idea there might be emotional games involved. I had just gone through a divorce three years earlier."

Despite Kathy's misgivings about getting romantically attached again, she continued to see Jerry as their long distance relationship continued. A few months later Jerry broke it off, however, saying he had to finalize his divorce with his third wife. Kathy agreed it was the best thing to do. She told Jerry that if he managed to get things straightened out, he could call her again.

About six months later Kathy got a call from Jerry's daughter, Christy. Kathy and she had become friends, partly because they lived closer together. Jerry was still in Phoenix, but his daughter Christy lived in Kentucky. Christy was secretly keeping Kathy informed about what Jerry was doing. She knew Kathy still hoped she would be with Jerry again. Christy called to invite Kathy for a weekend visit. Kathy accepted the invitation.

A few minutes later Christy called back and told Kathy, "I can't do this. I just can't do this."

Kathy said, "Can't do what?"

Christy admitted that Jerry wanted her to call, to set up a surprise meeting at her house with Kathy. "He really wants to meet you at my house," Christy said. "He wants to reconcile with you, and get back together with you."

Kathy said, "Oh really? Okay. But if he wants to reconcile with me, he can call me himself."

Kathy knew that she couldn't continue on only as Jerry's friend anymore. She couldn't be satisfied with that kind of relationship. Kathy thought Jerry, now divorced for six months, had had enough time. In Kathy's mind it was clear Jerry would have to make a choice. Either he wanted a relationship or not.

Jerry called her a few hours later.

Kathy was at work, where she answered the phone, "KJ Express. Can I help you?" KJ Express was the name of Kathy's delivery service. KJ stood for Kathryn Jean.

Jerry said, "I want a pizza delivery."

Kathy knew who it was. She said, "I don't deliver pizza any more. Who is this?"

"Come on, you know who this is," Jerry said.

"Yes," Kathy said. "And if you don't want anything that can be delivered, I'm busy!"

"I really want to talk to you," Jerry replied. "Would you come out to Christy's and meet me there this next weekend?"

"I'll think about it," Kathy answered. "I have another call on the line. I have to go." Kathy hung up the phone and smiled.

She called Jerry back a half hour later and said she would be there.

After not seeing each other for six months they met again at Christy's home in Kentucky.

Christy's brothers were there, too. "It was a really interesting time," she remembered. "Jerry hadn't seen all his kids together at the same time for years. Jerry's children were now all in their twenties. He also saw some of his grandchildren for the first time. So it was a gathering and a healing in a lot of different ways."

Later that day, Jerry asked Kathy to marry him. She said yes. The wedding was two months later at a chapel in Mesa, Arizona. Later, they also had a private ceremony on a beach near Rocky Point, Mexico.

Jerry's relationship with Kathy was something he had never experienced before. He said, "She was always encouraging me to dig deep within my soul to find my purpose in life. She was interested in the same things I found stimulating and wanted us to discover more together. There was no criticism or ridicule, only interest and encouragement. I had never experienced a relationship like this. It provided me inner strength to find out what this gift was about and how to best use it. No one in my life had ever played such a monumental role in my confidence and sense of well being.

"It was the first time that I had a relationship with someone who took it to the next level," Jerry continued. "She was always right there, a hundred percent. It was like, how can we do this together? Let me help."

For two months, the newlyweds still lived apart. She was running her delivery business in Nebraska, and he was still running his electronics repair shop in north Phoenix. Both businesses were doing well, but one had to give it up so their marriage could bloom.

One day, Jerry called her and asked, "How would you like to have a roommate?"

Kathy said sure. So Jerry sold his business and moved to Nebraska so they could be together.

Seven months later, Kathy accompanied Jerry as they guided their first trip together to Peru. But while she was gone, a woman Kathy had trusted to run her delivery business ended up wrecking it instead. Within just days, the woman had stopped deliveries, fired employees and defaulted on every contract. Upon returning to Nebraska after only a week, Kathy's business was destroyed. Kathy returned to Phoenix with Jerry a few weeks later. Together they opened a shop repairing high end musician's electronics equipment.

It was during this time, in late 1999, that Jerry decided to go public with his healing ability and did the story with FOX-10 News. More healing clients started to show up, but Jerry still wasn't charging a set fee for his services. He only asked for donations, if his clients had money to offer.

Later, the two decided they wanted to move to Peru and set up a clinic so Jerry could heal people full time. They had a financial backer for the project, but when the dot-com bull market collapsed, so did the funding for Jerry and Kathy's project. A few weeks later they were back in Phoenix, and Jerry was fixing electronics again. He hated it.

Eventually they had to give up the home they were living in because they couldn't afford the payments. They next moved into a one bedroom apartment in central Phoenix that was owned by a friend in California. It was very small, dark and cramped.

"Then he started getting a few calls from across the country about doing energy healing and classes," Kathy said. The stories Jerry had done for FOX-10 News had been distributed to other FOX stations across the country. Jerry started getting calls from everywhere.

"There were several calls from Florida," Kathy said. "I thought if we could coordinate these people we could provide classes and schedule healings. We would need to develop our material and determine prices. I knew how amazing Jerry is with people and knew if this were planned out well enough we could make a living. And I thought, why don't we just hit the road? Jerry could do some healings. We could do some classes, just go from city to city."

Jerry said, "Well, we're not doing too well here. I'm game. Let's just go."

So off they went, with most of their belongings in the back of a worn out 1985 Chevy Suburban. They dropped off some of their belongings at Kathy's mother's home in Nebraska and continued on.

The trip led to several awakening experiences for Jerry and Kathy but didn't lead to a lot of financial gain. The people they helped from Florida to Michigan were often kind enough to put up the Wills in their home or a condo for a few days. But much of their earnings were spent on travel expenses, including repairs to their old Chevy Suburban. After spending much of a miserable winter in Raleigh, North Carolina, they decided to return to Phoenix.

Within a month Jerry and Kathy returned to the electronics repair business in Phoenix. In the back of their shop on 7th Avenue, Jerry maintained a small healing room where he continued to see and treat clients.

They also made some money when Jerry agreed with Kathy's suggestion that he start teaching a class in energy healing. About a dozen people signed up for Jerry's first class, and FOX-10 News did another story about Jerry and his students. That led to more healings and more clients calling Jerry for help. The electronics business began to fade, but his healing business picked up.

Jerry still wasn't sure he and Kathy could make ends meet just by energy healing. Kathy had done a lot of work with herbal remedies and was selling them on the side. But could they make it without Jerry's repair business?

"I really didn't have that much faith in the fact I could do this and make ends meet," Jerry said. "I could see the tangibility of doing the electronics work. There was a cause and effect. You fix this, they take it, they're happy and you get paid. But with working as a healer it was different."

First of all, Jerry knew there was a stigmatism attached to healers who charged money for their services. "Anyone charging for their service as a healer was immediately criticized," he said. "Most psychics and 'New Agers' were operating on donations. It seemed to me they were happy to be poor, like not having money was a badge of honor for many of them. To me it seemed they were acting like martyrs. If you charged money, they thought something was wrong with you. The ones that did charge money were considered snooty or opportunists."

But many of the people who served as mentors for Jerry did have a set fee. "Frank Baranowski was charging, and he lived in a nice home," Jerry said. "Jan Ross was charging money; she had a nice home and a nice store. Doctor Richard Ireland had bodyguards, a chauffeur and a huge estate over in Scottsdale, and a place in Beverly Hills. I'm looking at all this and thinking there's something way out of balance here. These people who are in poverty consciousness must be where they want to be."

Jerry says Kathy was the key to his decision to jump into healing as his only full time source of income.

Kathy said, "Believe me. People spend three hundred dollars or more on a new purse. They will spend three hundred dollars to get their health back."

She took Jerry to a nearby mall, and they looked at the prices for purses and shoes. She said, "Look at how much these new purses are."

Kathy asked one of the salespeople if they sell many of them.

"Oh, yes," he said. "We sell them all the time."

"Three hundred bucks for a pair or shoes, or a purse," Jerry said. "I was amazed."

Kathy said, "When he saw how much money people were spending on shoes or a purse, I asked him, 'Isn't it worth two or three hundred dollars for them not to have their illness? How much would it be worth to them?'"

Within a month, Jerry ended the electronic repair business and redesigned the shop. Now it was dedicated to health, healing and teaching. Within a year they had set up a second clinic for healing inside a medical plaza in north Phoenix. They also started another round of healer classes. Because of Kathy's encouragement the standard fee for a healing session was set at three hundred dollars. Jerry still didn't turn away anyone who couldn't pay.

The north Phoenix healing clinic location didn't work out. Just before leaving on another Peru trip, the doctor who owned the complex asked Jerry to move out. She said some of her patients were complaining about Jerry and his wife smoking outside the building. Jerry suspected something more, but didn't pursue it.

After returning from Peru, Jerry and Kathy re-established their business inside the building where he once repaired electronics. And later he and Kathy hosted clients at a home they rented for a short time in Peoria, west of Phoenix.

Kathy's work with natural supplements complemented Jerry's. Many of Jerry's clients walked away healed, and with a supply of supplements Kathy developed to help them live a more healthy and drug free lifestyle.

"I've always been interested in herbal remedies, and what herbs can do," Kathy said. "When we were on the road, Jerry and I talked about how we could develop our own line of supplements and detoxification programs."

Kathy did extensive research, talked to a lot of people, and said she created a new line, building on what others had already discovered. "I investigated the different herbs and different elements you can put into a supplement. I looked at what others were doing, added my touch, and came up with my own unique formulations.

She doesn't sit down and talk with people about what they should eat. She said Jerry does that. But Jerry will ask them to talk to Kathy about what she can offer. "I don't counsel people about it," she said. "Jerry takes the information and tells them about it. I only offer my insight and knowledge if they ask."

But it's more than moral support Kathy offers Jerry, and it's more than the herbal supplements Kathy provides for their clients. Kathy also keeps things moving. She is the organizer in their business relationship. Kathy keeps the schedule organized, keeps the paperwork in order. She even helps Jerry plan and execute the trips to Peru they still offers through their "XpeditionsTV.com" website.

But Kathy remains in awe every time she sees Jerry heal someone.

"I don't know how it happens," she said. "But I know it has everything to do with the transfer of energy. It is just amazing to me."

Often asked about Jerry's healing abilities, Kathy finds it hard to describe. "It is heartwarming," Kathy said. "It's the feeling you get when you do something special for someone. You didn't realize it meant so much, or touched them so deeply, until they tell you how much it meant to them, how much they appreciated it."

As Jerry's fame grows, he has yet to see much fortune. He makes enough money to live, to eat and to buy some clothes, to pay the rent. But he won't be buying his own estate next to the late Richard Ireland's Scottsdale mansion anytime soon.

He has gained some famous friends and clients, however, including one very rich, very famous and successful Hollywood actress.

Chapter Eleven
Healing Hollywood

The phone rang one afternoon, and it was Hollywood on the other end. A woman we will call Jane (not her real name) was calling Jerry to see if he could come to Los Angeles and treat her roommate, who had pancreatic cancer.

She asked Jerry what he charged, and asked how soon he could fly out to see her. The sick woman couldn't fly, so Jerry would have to come to Los Angeles. "I told her what my fee would be," said Jerry. It was fifteen hundred dollars, plus airfare and hotel.

Jane said fine. She would have someone pick up Jerry at the airport, and Jerry could stay at her house while he was in Los Angeles.

Jerry agreed and said he could fly out to Los Angeles the next day.

A day later Jerry was in Los Angeles and Jane introduced him to her friend, Kay. "It was a very serious situation." Jerry said. " Kay looked like she had nothing wrong with her, and yet here she was being told that she had limited time left, and had to do something very fast."

A third woman who was there was another friend of Kay, and had helped to convince her to see Jerry.

She and Jane told Jerry that Kay was a bodyguard for a famous Hollywood actress (who will not be named in this book because she failed to respond to interview requests). Jane said she was also the producer for this actress.

Jerry wasn't too surprised. "I didn't know who I was dealing with, but I sometimes don't. It was no big deal."

With her friends watching, Jerry and Kay went out to the patio, and he prepared to begin. "Just as I am starting to work, and build up energy, these dogs they have start going nuts," Jerry said. Kay and Jane had several big dogs, including five or six boxers. "All the dogs are just crazy and jumping all over me. I'm trying to keep them away while I start working on her, but I can't." The dogs all want Jerry's attention. He had no idea why. "I tried to recompose myself. I was tired from flying. I was tired from all the travel. It was nine o'clock at night and they wanted me to do something, but I couldn't. Not with all those dogs jumping around."

To escape the dogs, Jerry and Kay moved inside and he began again. "I saw what was going on," Jerry said. "I started destroying it. I felt pretty good about it. The girl felt really tired and went off to bed. Of course, I instructed her to do just that, even if she wasn't tired."

The next day, Kay had an appointment with a Sufi healer. Apparently hedging her bets, she wanted to see another healer, too. Jerry and her two friends went along. They introduced Jerry to the Sufi healer at a New Age festival that was taking place in LA. "This man had a booth," Jerry said. "I was told he was a leader of the Sufi community in Los Angeles."

According to the website, all-natural.com, the Sufi healing method is an "Islamic healing method using Divine spiritual power practiced exclusively by the Sufis for centuries. The basic principle in Sufi healing is that the true healer is God Himself; the Sufis only act as mediators." Sufis in Pakistan and Indonesia are famous for piercing themselves with all kinds of sharp objects in the head or neck, and then healing themselves instantly. Many of their ceremonies have been videotaped and shown on different cable TV channels.

"After we were introduced," Jerry said, "he just stood there staring at me. I just stood there staring down at him."

The Sufi healer put his hands out on either side of Jerry's arms, and said, "It's really good to meet you. You are a very special person. You are needed very badly on this planet."

Jerry and the man then begin walking around the convention site. Kay and the man met later at the Sufi healer's center. The Sufi healer sat down with Kay and started to do his prayers. He suddenly stopped, looked up at her and said, "Jerry worked with you already, hasn't he?"

"Yes," Kay said.

"Then there is nothing I can do," the man said. "He's a much more powerful healer than I am. You should do as he says. Wait. And rest."

But according to Jerry it didn't end there. "Kay was seeing another woman, a long time friend who had recently started studying the Sufi healing method," he said.

The woman had already spent thousands of dollars to study Sufi healing with the Sufi healer Jerry met. "So the next day, this gal is giving Kay a Sufi healing session, but she is a novice; she doesn't know what she is doing, or undoing as it turned out," Jerry said. "Later that afternoon, this woman developed the exact same symptoms as Kay, and she became very ill."

What's worse is that the woman had undone everything Jerry had done for Kay. "She burst the bubble, to sort of speak," Jerry said. "She tampered with the energy I had put in place to destroy the cancer around her pancreas."

Now Kay felt horribly sick, too, and so did the woman who worked with her. Kay called Jerry and told him what had happened.

"You have to be kidding," Jerry said. "You didn't let her work on you, did you?"

Kay said, "Yes. She is studying to be a healer. I didn't think there would be any harm in it."

"Oh no," Jerry said. "Let me check out what is going on with you."

Jerry did, and he found out his work had been completely undone. "I tried to work on her again," he said. "But the field she had left was messed up so badly that it just wasn't happening."

264

When Jerry works on someone, it takes some period of time for a complete healing to take place. If the person Jerry works on has someone else work on them immediately afterwards, then it does something to disrupt the healing process. Jerry describes it as "breaking the spell."

Meanwhile, Jerry was still in Los Angeles, staying with Kay and Jane at their home. Jane told him that she'd been speaking with the actress she and Kay worked with. The actress was in New York, but she was hoping to meet Jerry.

"I can't go to New York," Jerry replied, "but it would be nice to meet her."

"You don't have to," Jane said. "It's her birthday tomorrow, and she's coming home. She wanted to know if you could stay over one more day to see her."

Jerry said, "Sure. No problem."

Jerry was supposed to fly back to Phoenix early the next morning, but he decided to stay. The first thing he did was to call Kathy to tell her he was staying.

The next afternoon, Jerry and Jane drove to the Beverly Hills home of the actress Jerry was about to meet. It was a huge house. "It was an amazing place but nothing I was used to being around. It was intimidating," Jerry said.

When the two walked in, the first thing Jerry saw was a huge room with several large windows. "You look out onto a pond with these huge goldfish in it," Jerry said. The view was spectacular. "You look over all these mountains and greenery, and you couldn't tell if there was anyone nearby. There might be another home right next door, but you could never tell."

Jerry strolled around a bit, and eventually came to the kitchen, "Which was as big as the house I'm living in," he said. "There were women in there. All of them were very busy putting together food trays and cooking. There was this closet with several large refrigerators filled with stacks and stacks of water and all kinds of drinks. There were large silver pots being filled with coffee. And these gals were walking around in little maid outfits. I thought the whole thing was comical, like in a movie. It didn't seem real. I'm just chuckling to myself, thinking. 'How strange is this!'"

Then people started to arrive, including the actress's brother and his girlfriend. Jane was the only person Jerry knew who was at the party. "Movie stars, producers and all these people are just wandering around," Jerry said. "I'm off to the side, or outside on the patio having a cigarette. I'm just sort of hanging back."

Then she arrived. Someone hollered, "She's here, she's here!"

Jerry went back inside with his cup of coffee and just stood there watching the scene unfold. He saw the actress, and thought right away that she wasn't as tall as he always thought she was. But no one ever is, he mused. They were always larger than life on the big screen.

Jerry was very impressed with her nonetheless. She looked beautiful. She was radiant. Not because he was thinking of her as a movie star. Jerry knew instantly that the actress was just a beautiful woman.

Like anyone would expect her to do, the actress worked the crowd, happily laughing with her guests about her birthday, and making sure everyone was having a good time. Jerry watched her closely. She was wearing blue jeans with a belt made of rope, and a t-shirt, nothing fancy, Jerry thought. She was giving people hugs and saying hello to them. She was also giving them kisses on the cheeks.

Jerry made a move toward the kitchen door so he could make a quick exit if he had to, because he was starting to feel a little nervous, and out of place.

But he continued to stand there, all alone, away from the crowd, trying not to be noticed. After greeting nearly everyone else in the room, the actress looked over at Jerry and smiled. She then nodded in his direction, and Jerry nodded back.

After about twenty more minutes of her greeting and talking to all of her guests, Jerry drifted away to get another cup of coffee. He also grabbed some sort of cake that was put out for her guests. It was the best cake Jerry had ever tasted.

Suddenly a voice said, "I've heard a lot about you." It was the actress and she was standing right next to him.

Jerry nervously laughed, and said, "I've heard a lot about you. In fact, I've seen some of your movies."

She laughed, and replied, "Yeah? You and about a million other people."

"Okay," Jerry said. "I'm feeling all shaky inside because you are this movie star person. I'm not really prepared to have a colorful conversation with you at this point in time because I don't really know what to say. And I don't want to sound stupid."

She smiled at Jerry and seemed to understand.

"So all I can say," Jerry continued, "is that it's really a pleasure to meet you and thank you for your hospitality and for allowing me into your home."

"Well, I've heard a lot about you," she said. "And what I've heard is that you are quite an amazing person. I'd like to know more, but it's going to have to wait until I get rid of all these people. But when they go home, I'd like to spend some time with you. I have a problem," she continued, "and I'd like to see if you can help me with it."

"Yes, of course," Jerry said. "No problem at all. I'm quite comfortable here. I'll just go out and have a cigarette and relax."

"You make yourself at home," she said. "Just tell one of the servers if you want anything at all, or come and get me, and I'll make sure you are taken care of."

After that, she went back to her guests.

Jerry went outside with his coffee and had another cigarette. At least that was over, he thought. Now he could relax and wait for her party to end.

Jerry did get to chat a while with her brother and his girlfriend. He also got to spend some time with another actor, this one a famous comedian. "He was funny as hell," Jerry said. "Oh my God, was he funny. We were going back and forth like Dean Martin and Jerry Lewis. He would say something, and I'd come right in with something else. We were just laughing and laughing, and people were laughing…He is very witty and a very nice person. I really enjoyed that time laughing with him."

Jerry said it wasn't until about eleven o'clock at night that everyone had left, except for himself and the movie star's producer, Jane. Even the hired help had finally cleared out.

The actress came up to Jerry and asked, "Where shall we do this?"

Jerry looked around, but it was such a huge house he wasn't sure where would be the best place to begin. "Where in the house are you the most comfortable?" Jerry asked.

"I'm most comfortable in my bedroom, I guess," she replied. "It's my sanctuary."

"Fine," Jerry said. "Let's go to your bedroom and do the work there."

Jerry, the actress, and Jane headed upstairs to her bedroom. First they walked through a large office at the top of the stairs. Jerry looked at ceilings that were at least twenty feet tall. He couldn't believe he was actually inside a Beverly Hills mansion.

Her bedroom was through the other side of the office. The room was almost as big as the room downstairs where she met her guests. But the furniture seemed simple by comparison. She had just a small bed and some chairs, nothing special.

Jerry did see a little place to the side where she had set up a small Buddhist shrine. A practicing Buddhist, her shrine was simple with a small Buddha and a prayer rug.

"Okay. Do what you need to do in order to become centered. Bring a deep peace and a sense of spiritual energy into yourself," Jerry told her.

She went over to her altar and began to meditate. As Jerry watched, she spread out a piece of cloth on the floor and kneeled down in front of Buddha.

When she finished, she said to Jerry, "Okay. I'm ready. Do you want me to lie on the bed?"

Jerry said, "No. All I really need are two chairs."

The actress and Jane moved two small chairs to the side of the room near the bed. Jerry sat in one, the actress in the other, and they faced each other.

"I've been filming a movie," she told Jerry. "And the producers are starting to notice that I have problems." She told Jerry that she was showing signs of Bell's Palsy. She couldn't see out of her right eye very well. She could hardly hear out of her right ear. She was very afraid that she was going to be in big trouble because it was getting worse and worse.

Like he had done in every healing, Jerry took her hands and started to concentrate. He immediately found several problems. Standing slightly behind and beside her right side, Jerry placed his hands on the side of her head and focused. One by one each area was addressed until Jerry felt the conditions had been resolved. A few minutes later, Jerry asked, "Look at me."

She opened her eyes.

"Now, look around the room," Jerry said.

Jane was sitting on the bed nearby. The actress looked over towards her, and then looked around the room.

She then put her hand over one eye and looked around. She said, "Oh my God. I can see."

She then gasped, and said, "Say something! Say something!"

Jerry said, "Can you hear me all right?"

"My hearing is back!" She then touched her face. "It's not numb anymore. I can feel my face!"

271

Looking into a mirror it was obvious to the actress her face had changed slightly. The woman was clearly amazed. "It worked, it worked!" she said. She also started crying her eyes out. Then she got up and gave Jerry a big hug and a kiss on the cheek. "Oh my God," she said. "I can't believe this!"

A moment later, one of the maids came into the room and told Jane that someone else was there to see the actress. It was her masseuse to give her a massage before going to bed.

"Here's the deal," Jerry said. "I don't want anybody messing with your energy for at least two days. You just stay here. You just relax, you decompress, and you finish healing." Jerry continued, "If someone is going to put their hands on you, I need to know right now so I can modify what I've done so maybe that can be done without hurting you."

"Hey, I'll do whatever you tell me to do." She then told her maid to send the masseuse home.

After thanking him again, Jerry and Jane left.

As they headed home, Jane said, "Wow, you made quite an impression on her."

"Yes," Jerry said. "I guess that would make quite an impression, wouldn't it?"

They returned to Kay and Jane's home about midnight.

The next day Jerry had to catch his flight home, but he and Jane stopped at the movie star's home one more time so he could look in on her.

The woman was bubbly and laughing away, delighted with how she felt. She said, "I have to show you something. In this movie I have to do all these kicks, and I'd like to kick up to your shoulder."

"Sure," Jerry said.

She explained she had been practicing for awhile, but when she first reported problems to her doctor, they had examined her by inserting a tube up an artery in her leg. She hadn't been able to kick since the exam, and she didn't want to tell the movie producers about it. She said she had been fudging it.

"But now watch," she told Jerry as she demonstrated several kicks and Karate -like moves, without any pain.

"What do you think of that?" she asked Jerry.

"Wow. That's just like in the movies!" Jerry said. He was pleased that she seemed so happy.

"If you ever need anything, all you have to do is let me know," she said. She then asked Jerry how much he had charged for his visit to LA.

"Fifteen hundred dollars," he told her.

She laughed. "If I had known you could do this, I would have paid ten times that amount."

"It's just how I make ends meet," Jerry said as he shrugged his shoulders.

"You have no idea, Jerry, what people would pay around here to have access to you. You could write your own ticket," she said. "How many millions of dollars do you want to make this year?"

Jerry said he hadn't really given it much thought. "I was thinking more in terms of being able to afford the rent and my car payment."

"You have to grow up and join the real world." She then said she had paid the fifteen hundred dollars for him to see her bodyguard, Kay. "If I had any idea that you could do what you just did for me, what you've charged is nothing. I know people who are worth billions of dollars, and if they or a family member have a problem, all you would have to do is go in and do your work, and they would give you a million dollars, whatever you ask."

She asked for Jerry's phone number, and he gave it to her.

"All you have to do is have them give me a call," Jerry said. "But it's not really about the money, it's about helping people. If I can just help people, then that is a really good thing. The money part of it...sure, everyone wants to have some money. But I'm not really doing it because I want a lot."

The woman said she thought that was the right thing to say, but Jerry wasn't sure if she was convinced.

She asked Jerry if there was anything else she could do. Jerry thought for a moment, and said, "Well, I have this really good friend in Phoenix. He's not going to know what to think if he gets a phone call from you."

"Who is he?" she asked.

"Rod Haberer. He's a news producer for Fox TV, a really nice guy. And I think it would be a real treat for him. He's a big fan of yours."

What Jerry didn't say was that he had called Rod the night before and told him about working with this famous actress. Rod accused Jerry of pulling his leg, but Jerry insisted he was telling the truth and would prove it.

That next day in Beverly Hills, the actress told Jerry, "Sure, what's his number?"

Jerry gave her Rod's phone number at FOX-10, and she called. Unfortunately, he was not at his desk, and she got Rod's voice mail instead.

"I got his voice mail," she told Jerry.

"Damn." Jerry was disappointed he wasn't there.

"I'll leave him a message." She paused a moment as the recorded greeting ended. "Hello, Rod. This is (her name). I'm here with Jerry Wills, and I'm calling just to say…." Then she made a noise common with school children pretending to pass gas, sometimes called "the raspberries." In the background, Jerry was laughing hysterically. Then she hung up the phone.

After hanging up on Rod's voice mail, the actress turned to Jerry and said, "You tell him the next time I call to answer the damn phone."

Jerry laughed again. "He probably still won't believe me. But once he gets that message he's going to be thinking about the next phone call that comes in. He'll never know who might be calling." They both had a good laugh.

It was time for Jerry to go. He said goodbye, and she gave him another kiss on the cheek, along with a big hug. "I've got a guest house down here being fixed up," she said. "If you come to LA and you need a place to stay, you can stay here at my home or in the guest house. Or if you need a place to work out of, you can work out of the guest house. Just let me know."

She also said she had to get Jerry on "Oprah," that Oprah was a good friend of hers.

Jerry said that would be pretty awesome. He then thanked her again, and he and Jane left for the airport.

"Funny thing is," Jerry said later, "she was on 'Oprah,' and talked about her medical problems, but she never mentioned me."

The actress went on to finish working on her movie, doing all her own stunts. Jerry never got another call from her.

It is worth noting that the author of this book tried to reach the actress several times through her producer Jane to ask about the encounter with Jerry. Jane said she knew all about Jerry, but there has been no response to interview requests by the time this book was written.

Maybe her encounter with Jerry Wills is something the actress will never admit to publicly. Maybe being cured by an energy healer is not something she wants to talk about. If not today, maybe someday she will. Energy Healing is apparently still something that gains acceptance only slowly – apparently even in the land of make-believe.

Chapter Twelve
The Healer in Peru

Jerry's trip to Peru in June and July of 2005 was anything but ordinary. It started innocently enough. Jerry had a group of about eighteen tourists on his usual ten day trip, with the three day Marcahuasi extension for those who were interested. But this time, Jerry had agreed to help guide a larger group of people right after his trip wrapped up. His friend, Thomas Morton, had signed up two busloads of people from the Association for Research and Enlightenment.

"He had about fifty-six people signed up, and it was a challenge," Jerry said. "They were a group of forty to fifty-plus year olds, having a blast and acting like teenagers. We had a seriously dedicated schedule and I was supposed to help make certain everyone was at the right place as we progressed through the trip. Often, small groups would wander off to look at something they thought was interesting, and I would have to find them. It was demanding for me to work with so many different types of personalities. To keep everyone in tow, they had to be corralled. When you are that age, you have your likes and dislikes. Most never traveled through a third world country. Services and standards are different in Peru. As a result, there were those who had a habit of complaining about things that weren't to their liking. Some didn't like the fact they didn't have a soft, comfortable bed or food to their satisfaction. It was a real challenge, and a two week period I was feeling some anxiety about."

On the drive down to Nazca, the group was separated into two busses. In one bus, Thomas had his laptop computer, and he started showing passengers video news clips about Jerry, the ones aired by FOX-10 in Phoenix. The people who saw the videos were amazed. No one knew much about Jerry or that he was a healer. They only considered him one of their tour guides

About halfway to Nazca, which is an eight-hour drive from Lima, Jerry and Thomas switched busses, and Thomas proceeded to show everyone on the other bus the same news stories about Jerry. Now, everyone was really curious about one of their hosts. But at first, none of them came forward to ask Jerry about his healing gifts.

Then something happened. An older lady stubbed her big toe pretty badly, and was in a lot of pain. She was hobbling around telling everyone how she hurt it so bad that she thought it was broken.

That next morning, before leaving the hotel, the woman came to see Jerry. It was five-thirty in the morning and Jerry was having a cup of coffee and a cigarette, trying to get his brain going because he is not a morning person.

"I heard you're a healer," she said. "I hurt my toe really bad, and I'm afraid for the rest of this trip I'm going to be laid up with this thing. I've had this before, and it just doesn't heal."

Jerry looked across the table at the woman. She was clearly in pain and seemed a little embarrassed asking for his help. She obviously could see that Jerry was struggling to wake up. Jerry downed the last bit of his coffee, put out his cigarette and asked, "Would you like me to help you?"

"Yes," she said, limping towards a nearby chair.

"Okay, sit down and let me take a look."

The woman sat in the chair next to Jerry and held up her foot.

Jerry closed his eyes and put his hand around her toes. He saw the problem right away. She had dislocated her big toe. Her connective tissue wasn't as strong as it should have been. So Jerry strengthened the tissue around the toe, repaired the damage and left it with enough energy to heal rapidly.

When Jerry was finished, he said, "All right. Stand up now. Tell me how it feels."

The woman slowly stood and gingerly put some weight on her bad foot.

"Oh my Lord," she said.

"Is it better?"

"Yes. Much."

Jerry said, "Look, it's going to be a little sore for the next six hours or so. But that will just work itself away, and by this time tomorrow you will be fine. Just don't go jamming your toe again. Please watch where you are walking."

"Okay," the woman said, as she took out her checkbook and wrote a three-hundred dollar check to Jerry. Jerry thanked her and tried to ready himself for what was sure to be a long day.

It was about to get longer, because within twenty-four hours, the woman had told everyone on the tour what Jerry had done for her. Soon everyone knew about him, and people started noticing that she wasn't limping anymore. The word "healer" spread like wildfire throughout the large tour group. By the time they got back to the hotel, which was nearly a full day later, other people started asking Jerry if he could help them. They asked how much he charged. He told them, and no one seemed to have a problem with it.

"It was starting to get out of hand, all these people talking to me and paying less attention to the Peruvian tour guides," Jerry said. "So the next day, while I was on one bus, I sent out a piece of paper that said if you want to have a session with me, write your name down. It went all the way through both busses, and I had about thirty-five people sign up."

Most of the people Jerry worked on were astonished, and had instant results. Some did not. "This one guy had taken Viagra, and it caused a blood vessel in his eye to burst. He couldn't see," Jerry explained. "I did the best I could, and I said it will take some time for your vision to come back.

Later he was starting to see some light and some patterns, though his vision never returned completely."

Others had even bigger problems. "There were a couple of others who had some pretty serious things going on, oddball things that take some time, more time than I was able to give them on the trip." One of his new clients had a serious blood toxicity problem. "It was going to take her a year or more to get out of that," he said. "But by and large, most people just had a variety of aches and pains, and I was able to help them."

One success that stood out for Jerry was his work with Joe Overly from Sullivan, Missouri.

When Jerry first met him, Joe didn't seem very open or friendly. But when Jerry passed his paper around for people who wanted to see him, Joe's name was at the top of the list.

"He didn't say much on the trip," Jerry remembered. "He didn't say much to anybody. His wife was a nurse, and they were just off by themselves going through the trip, not standing out in any way." But Jerry thought to himself that Joe looked sad, "Like he was grumpy and unhappy. He just didn't look like a happy person. People didn't talk to him because he looked like he was on the verge of being pissed off." Jerry didn't think that was really the case with Joe, but he just didn't know what was bothering him, until he signed up to be treated.

They were at the St. Augustine Hotel in the Sacred Valley near Cuzco, when it was Joe's turn to visit Jerry. "I didn't take them in the order they were written down," Jerry said. "I just took them as I could. It was busy all the time. I'm just seeing people in the middle of the night, between stops, whenever I can. It was just crazy."

Jerry went to Joe's room at about nine o'clock at night, after a long day touring Peru through the Sacred Valley. Joe and his wife Joy were there to greet him.

Joe told Jerry about his arm. "He had been working at home doing something, and had a stroke," Jerry said. "That basically left him as a consciousness in a body that didn't work. He didn't have anything wrong with him before that."

Joy said that her husband had gone through hell for a couple of years. Physical therapy and painful rehabilitation brought him back to a point. But he lived with excruciating pain and weakness in his right arm that never went away.

He told Jerry that he couldn't even turn a key in a locked door knob. He couldn't hold his arm up long enough to put the key in.

On top of everything else, doctors told Joe just prior to the trip that he had prostate cancer. He told Jerry they had done fifteen or twenty biopsies on him, and one of them came back suspicious.

"Well, if it's suspicious one out of twenty, they have to say you have prostate cancer, but you probably don't," Jerry said to Joe.

But Joe said he was still really concerned about that.

Jerry could see in his face that he was absolutely terrorized. "I don't know if you have prostate cancer or not," Jerry said. "But let's take a look."

As usual Jerry prepared himself, then began to examine what was wrong with Joe. Because Jerry was in Peru, and interference with the outside world is so minimal, he can tap into his abilities much more profoundly.

Jerry said, "Stand up for a second."

Joe stood.

Jerry put one hand on Joe's stomach, another on his back. He didn't see any cancer. "Joe, I don't see any cancer," he said. "I think they're feeding you a line. You look like a meal ticket to me. I think you'd better have someone else check this before you do anything."

"Okay," Joe said, looking at least a little relieved.

"I'll throw some energy into the prostate and try to resolve any issues you have there, but I don't see any cancer."

Jerry was annoyed by the whole thing. "This really ticks me off," Jerry told Joe and his wife. "You have all these things happening, and now this? I don't think this is God's plan for you."

"I really don't think so either," Joe said.

Joe again asked Jerry about his arm. "If I could just use my arm again, I'd be happy," he said.

285

"Oh, that's nothing," Jerry replied. Jerry placed both hands on Joe's arm and went back to work.

After a few moments, Jerry said, "Try moving your arm."

Joe raised it without any pain. "Look, honey!" he said.

"There you go," Jerry said as Joe swung his arm around pain free and laughed. "It might be stiff for a day or so, so don't overdo it."

"I won't," Joe said. "It feels wonderful. Thank you."

The next morning, Jerry was in the crowded restaurant attached to the hotel with the other fifty or so guests. Joe and Joy were one of the last to arrive for breakfast. Before sitting at their table, Joe held up his arm and started swinging it around. "Look, Jerry," he yelled over to him, "There's nothing wrong!"

"All these other people were watching," Jerry told me. "And they're all thinking, 'I want some of that.' From that point on, Joe was the life of the party. And they all thoroughly enjoyed the moment."

"It was so bad," Joe said later, "I couldn't turn a key in the lock, and I couldn't turn the knob on the door to open it. Jerry worked on me, and I can tell you it is fantastic. It's really great."

Joe had a huge smile on his face. "Jerry, thank you a million. God bless."

His wife Joy was also impressed by the healing. "Jerry is such a wonderful person," she said. "He has a real gift, a gift from God. We were very blessed to meet him."

When they returned home to Sullivan, Missouri, Joe tried to have the test results on his prostate re-checked. But the doctors wouldn't do it.

Joy said they decided to have her husband's prostate treated anyway, so they did. And Joe is now cancer free. Whether it was Jerry's work or the doctor's treatment that cured Joe is impossible to tell. But Joe is sure Jerry played a big part.

Back in Peru, the list of people requesting Jerry's services continued to grow, especially after he worked on Joe.

Another person who signed up to see Jerry was Luisa Santamaria, a fifty-five-year-old registered nurse from New York City. She was also a member of the Association for Research and Enlightenment, the main group taking part in the tour Jerry and his friend were guiding.

Luisa had a bad knee after injuring it seventeen years before, and knew she would have a hard time getting around while on the Peru expedition. "I gave it a lot of thought about even attempting this trip because I knew there would be a lot of stairs," she said afterwards. "I really prepared as much as I could with swimming, which was the perfect exercise for me. I swam as much as I could as I tried to get in shape. But I had to be careful. If I overdid it, then I would be in pain."

Being a registered nurse, Luisa knew the problems with her knee could be corrected by surgery. But she wanted to try other therapies first.

"I'd been to physical therapy. And I'd been to other healers, and some were very helpful," she said.

While in Peru, and after hearing about Jerry's abilities, she decided to give him a try.

She said it went very well. "I was amazed," she said. "He just worked with breathing at first. Then he put his hands on my knee. Then I walked around a few times and tried it out in front of him. And it was totally healed. I was pain free for the first time in seventeen years."

Luisa can understand people having doubts about healers like Jerry. After all, she is a registered nurse, and even she had her doubts. "But I know this was an incredible healing," she said. "It's not that I don't go to doctors; I do. I mean, if I had a broken bone, I would have gone to a doctor. But this was a soft tissue problem, and I knew from experience it wasn't something easily treated. It was treated conventionally, and it didn't work that well."

But after seeing Jerry, her knee pain vanished. "I think Jerry is really phenomenal. I really do," she said.

By the time the trip was over, Jerry had worked on thirty-six people, and had earned some extra money. No one had balked at his $300.00 fee. "I didn't feel at all uncomfortable paying him whatever he asked," Luisa said. "I have a sense that he is someone who uses his money wisely, and it's not just to have a lot of luxuries in his life. I've always felt that Jerry supports people in ways that are his own business, but my sense is this money goes to help others, not just Jerry. Because that's the kind of man he is."

Going to Peru is one way Jerry made money, mostly as a tour guide. But each time he visits Peru he is enriched in other ways as well, usually by the visits and experiences he shares with the local shamen. After years of interaction with the Peruvian medicine men, most now consider Jerry one of them.

The secret, Jerry said, is learning to listen. "I've learned a lot of things," he said. "But mostly to just shut up and listen. That is what they are all about. They have this macho thing down there. They have the knowledge and you do not, so shut up and hold on...although they don't say that. But if you don't shut up, they will not let you know what you want to know."

Jerry finds each shaman he meets very interesting. "Their talents manifest in a variety of ways," he said, "Either with their apparent sorcery with indigenous plants, or with their other customs and practices. They have a tendency to be real tricksters, but they only do it to find out how real you are. Then they aren't interested in tricking you anymore because it's a waste of their time. They just enjoy putting you through the grinder to find out who you are and what you are all about. Once they figure it out, and they like you, they spend time with you."

Jerry has asked them for help, especially when it comes to their knowledge of medicinal plants and how to use them to create natural remedies. "I've learned a lot from shamen by being a part of their ceremonies and watching what they do. They also teach me how to work with plants, how to make this potion or this tea they are making for some ailment. They have also shown me how they go about looking over a person and how they come up with a treatment."

Jerry said he soon learned what the shamen do is not that different from his own approach to healing. "It's pretty general stuff," he said. "It's not that different from what I do. It's just that their perspectives are different because they grew up in the jungle where this knowledge has been passed down for hundreds of generations."

Jerry said the knowledge all shamen gain is passed down from father to son. "Rarely does it go to a woman, and it only goes to one son, chosen by the grandfather because the grandson shows that he wants to learn." If the child refuses to become a shaman, the family picks another son. "Up until about thirty to forty years ago, it was traditional to accept the knowledge. It was a badge of honor. With the encroachment of civilization into their jungle world, they are losing some of that now."

Shamen that Jerry knows are typically not very young. Some of them look younger than their years because of the healing knowledge they possess. "They are very skilled in what they do," Jerry said. "It doesn't mean that they are flawless and have all the answers all the time. They do the best with what they've got, and sometimes they miss the mark." Jerry admits the same thing happens to him, but not often.

It's that honesty, and Jerry's own healing talents, that allowed shamen to welcome Jerry as one of them. "Because I was sincerely interested in what they do, and I bugged them so much because I wanted to know more, they accepted me. They developed a sense of respect for me because of willingness to learn and my persistence."

Jerry's charity has also helped. "They have all seen or heard about my trips into villages to bring needed items, food or medicines when needed." While in Peru, Jerry and Kathy do their best to help those in need, especially when they see children suffering. "If the children need something like clothes, shoes, or maybe a dentist, we try to help them as much as we can."

Shamen also allow Jerry to use his special gift to help native people. "That is how I got this necklace," Jerry said as he pointed to a beautiful necklace he says is made of bone and conch that was hand woven thousands of years ago. "It belonged to a healer who died centuries ago and has now been passed down to me."

Jerry said Peruvian shamen have developed a respect for him that he deeply appreciates. "And that respect has put me into a privileged association with them that allows me a bit more freedom than most others within their ranks," he said. "I can ask questions and get answers that I know I can trust, whereas a lot of folks who don't have that affiliation might ask questions and get answers, but they are just being told something to shut them up."

Jerry appreciates the help he gets from the native healers in Peru, but he knows they don't tell him everything. "Shamen have traditions that are passed down from generation to generation, and they know a lot," he said. "I've been able to glean quite a bit from my experiences with them, but I know it's just the tip of the iceberg, because they live it everyday."

Like shamen have done for him, Jerry also tries to pass down what he has learned. After all, shamen themselves might not be around much longer. "There may be people like myself who attempt to fill their shoes in one way or another," Jerry said. "But I don't think there will be individuals of their caliber a hundred years from now. They are on the way out."

Still, Jerry does what he can. One way to pass on their knowledge also proves to be one way Jerry can help himself make a living as a healer full time. From time to time he conducts a class in the mechanics of consciousness – the key to developing skills as an energy healer. As you will soon read, being a healer isn't only limited to those born with the ability. It is something Jerry believes he can teach, and something his students can learn.

Chapter Thirteen
The Mechanics of Consciousness

When Jerry started traveling the world over to talk about healing, he developed a one-day twelve-hour class to teach to those interested in learning more about what he could do, and what he had learned from Peruvian shamen. But after setting up shop in Phoenix as a full-time energy healer (and part-time Peruvian guide) he developed a six-part class in which he would instruct a small group of people over a six month period the skills necessary to become a healer. He called his class "The Mechanics of Consciousness."

He began teaching to groups of ten to twelve people. And at $85.00 per person per session, it turned out to be another way Jerry could make money as a healer, and pay the rent.

No one who signed up for the six sessions complained about the money. They were mostly well educated, well motivated people who knew that there had to be something beyond western medicine to cure the ills of the world. They hoped to find their answer by taking Jerry's class.

Jerry told all perspective students that his class was for the evolving spiritual warrior, "Who one day," Jerry wrote on his website, "may be sought out by those who desperately seek answers."

Jerry cites examples of past spiritual warriors. "As during ages ago," he writes, "when

Viracocha traveled to South America, or Quetzacotal wandered Central America, these individuals provided the remaining inhabitants of Earth with science, philosophy, mathematics and spiritual guidance. These were great healers and amazing warriors. They returned the knowledge to the people, defended the weak, assisted the infirmed and provided safe haven and comfort for the young. These incredible spiritual masters brought light to the world. As you progress through these courses, you will discover their training and yours are similar."

When Jerry's "spiritual warriors" met for the first time, they were assembled in what used to be Jerry's electronics repair shop. Now painted a yellow and orange pastel, with all kinds of artwork from Peru hanging on the wall, along with a few paintings done locally just for Jerry (Some are beautifully produced works by Phoenix artist Bill Foss), the room was just big enough for the dozen or so people who met there once a month for the next six months. Some were people Jerry had worked on before and they wanted to know more about what he does. Some of the people there were medical professionals, and one was a doctor.

Jerry, dressed as usual in extreme casualness, wore a colorful shirt, hiking shorts and sandals. His long hair was pulled back in a ponytail, and he sat before a colorful piece of artwork that looked like a large multi-colored circle.

"You are about to embark upon a journey into consciousness," Jerry told his students. "But beyond that it is going to be a journey into awareness, an expanded level of awareness which I am pretty certain everyone here is interested in achieving."

Jerry began by telling them about a recent drive he had from Flagstaff, Arizona, to Phoenix. In the middle of the night, a truck had rolled and crashed. When Jerry drove up to the accident scene, the driver was hanging upside down out of the overturned cab. He was bloodied and bruised by the accident and was clearly in bad shape. Jerry said he rushed over to the man, and with a few simple things, was "able to resolve some issues that were going to change his life in a very powerful way." When emergency medics finally arrived, they treated a man who seemed amazingly healthy for someone who had just bounced around inside an overturned truck cab.

"He didn't even know that I did it," Jerry said. "In an emergency situation, you do the best you can."

Jerry told his students a class like the one they were taking would give them that ability, "because you will know that you can do it, and you'll feel very comfortable using your talents to do something of this nature."

Jerry explained that not all of them would achieve the kind of success he has had, especially in the public arena. In fact success as a healer wasn't the sole reason for teaching the class. "The class is something you can derive information from that will enable you to, in you own life and in your own ways, develop healing techniques that provide you a sense of certainty you might not have had before."

Why does Jerry teach the class? He says he wants to show other people that they have the same skills, that healing isn't a peculiarity of his. He wants to show others than anyone can do it, they just need the knowledge.

Unlike magicians or maybe other healers or psychics, Jerry is willing to share his gift with others. It's not something he feels he must keep secret.

As his first session continued, Jerry explained to his students what he can do as a healer. "I have the ability to reorganize human tissue and turn it to jelly, and then I re-manifest it back into what it's supposed to be. I take things apart and I put them back together again. Sometimes I can go through it in just a half hour or so. Sometimes I have to see a person several times because the damage is so severe." And in a very honest admission, Jerry added, "Sometimes it doesn't work at all."

Jerry also cautioned, "I can't interfere with free will." And he led a discussion about what Jerry calls "Spiritual Ethics." "In a nutshell," he said, "do no harm, be kind, and listen." Adding, "You don't want to interfere with God's will, and you don't want to interfere with the path of another." Jerry said he always asks permission before doing a healing.

Referring back to the accident, Jerry admitted that sometimes a decision has to be made for someone who can't give his or her permission. "If there's someone who's been in an accident and they're mentally incapable and there is no time, then it's up to you to make a decision about what you are going to do."

And what does he mean by "God's will"? Jerry said he will sometimes bump into someone, or shake someone's hand, and he instantly sees something terribly wrong with that person. "But I don't say anything," he said. "The reason is: it doesn't serve God's plan. If this is happening and God wants me to be involved, then it will work itself out to where they'll be brought before me, and I'll help in whatever way that I can."

The discussion then turned to Jerry's thoughts on God. It provided some fascinating insight into Jerry's thinking about God and our own lives.

Jerry began by asking his students what their concept of God was. "Is God a man in a white beard?"

He brought up an eastern philosophy called Zen. One of the tenets of Zen, Jerry said, "is simplicity. God is considered to be the un-carved block of stone." (Remember the small stone of alabaster Jerry found on a railroad track in Peru?) He then asked the question, "What if there was no

299

God? What if God doesn't exist? What are the ramifications of that? What if this is all there is?"

His students had quizzical looks on their faces. Some looked disturbed.

Jerry went on. "If this was actually the case, and I'm not saying it is, would you feel empty and lost?"

Then he asked, "What is your relationship with you? How honest is it? How deep does it go?" Jerry said he wanted his students to look at themselves in the mirror, to strip away all the things they've heard about themselves from others, and be at peace with themselves because, "if there was no God, what is it that you have become but God? And if that is the case, how truthful are you being to yourselves about who you truly are, and how do you see yourselves in the moment when no one is looking except you?"

Jerry explained he strongly believes that "God lives within you, and what is God but the power of creation? And what are you doing? You are creating yourselves into a more brilliant image of what creation may actually offer and what the potentialities may actually be. You are looking for that moment when you understand how this feels to merge into what I call Divine awareness. You can almost feel how potent it is to control your destiny, to reach out and manifest the next moment. The desire to create has been and continues to flow through you like a warmth rushing through your body. God lives within you, but if you are going to find that point where you step into this role you need to see yourself clearly. The filters you've been provided by others were only meant to help them feel comfortable, safe or secure while they were near you. You now must find yourself. To do this requires you take a bold step and risk everything. It's time to remove the mask you've grown comfortable wearing, Take a long look at yourself and then bravely return to the world."

"When you see yourself," Jerry continued, "in an honest light, the first thing you see are your flaws because that's what you've been taught to look for. But more importantly, if you take a look and practice seeing what is right with who you are, without any judgment, you're not going to see those illusionary flaws. With practice and determination you slowly rediscover the beauty and presence of YOU. A being created perfect in the eyes of God, a divine aspect of the presence of creation. A person who is no longer limited by their fears, doubts or apprehensions of being an outcast because they dared to be themselves."

Jerry gave his students an assignment. "What I'd like you to do is take a look at yourself and try to suspend judgment," he told them. "Suspend judgment and see yourself in the light of truth, of you being an example of God walking on Earth."

"This is the living God within you acknowledging your existence, and this is you acknowledging the presence of God living here within every cell of your body. Try to feel and connect with this concept and presence. The more you become used to this feeling, this connection, the closer you are to understanding your role in creation. And the closer you become to being a part of the process of creation. This is what you were born to know and use to the benefit of yourselves and those who struggle to create."

The discussion on God ends, and Jerry moved on to more Earthly matters. He gave his students a lesson on breathing. And he wanted them to study ancient philosophical writings on medical ethics: heavy stuff for just the first month. His students didn't ask a lot of questions. They had a lot to consider.

About a month later, the class met again. Jerry took his customary place with his back to a wall that was painted pastel orange, but this time there was a white board behind him.

Jerry started this class by holding up a bottle of something he called a topical skin cancer treatment. It was a small eyedropper sized bottle, with a murky liquid inside. Jerry said it was a natural ointment that is applied directly to any form of skin cancer. "What it does," Jerry said, as he passed the bottle to the student next to him, "is absorb into the cancer. It travels down through the tiny fibers and cells that have changed, and it destroys it. It is made from Bloodroot using an old Indian formula handed down over the past few hundred years. The AMA and FDA has now made this formulation illegal to sell. However, the formula is available on the internet and it is not illegal if you make some for yourself.

Jerry also told his students where to go on his website if they wanted to see very graphic examples of how it works. "The area you treat becomes large, red, and inflamed. It looks infected. It gets very pussy and quite exaggerated. It looks as if something is very seriously wrong. Then it just dries up and the scab falls off. All of this happens within a couple of weeks. All that's left is a hole. You put some vitamin E oil on it, or something similar, and the skin regenerates itself. Once you are done, there isn't any evidence that anything was ever there."

Jerry used it as an example of alternative forms of healing that Western medicine had ignored. There were other examples as well.

Next, Jerry previewed their trip to Peru, the final phase of the class. He described a ceremony they might all want to take part in. "In order to gain a deeper understanding of those energies you experience an opportunity is available for you to join a shamanic ritual called the Ayahuasca ceremony." Jerry said those who choose to participate will meet in the jungle to drink Ayahuasca, which will send them on a spiritual journey.

But first, to get the full extent of the Ayahuasca experience, they should cleanse their bodies of toxins and begin to eat healthy food.

Jerry suggested they explore the possibility of a liver cleanse before drinking the Ayahuasca.

"As a healer," Jerry said, "I frequently see those who have problems with years of toxins in their systems. Their complications are due specifically to the amalgam in their teeth, or the pesticides they've ingested, or the cleaners used on their cars; it's all been absorbed into their systems. We are exposed to a lot of stuff. So if you do a liver cleanse prior to going to Peru, you are going to find that your journeys will be much more dynamic and you feel phenomenal."

What is this ancient concoction that will send people on a spiritual journey? Martin A. Lee, author of The Beast Reawakens and Acid Dreams: The CIA, LSD and the Sixties Rebellion, writes that Ayahuasca is a fearsome, foul tasting jungle brew sold by the liter.

"The word is from the Quechua language; it means 'vine of the soul,' 'vine of the dead,' or 'the vision vine,'" he writes. "This legendary industrial-strength hallucinogen is used…to heal the sick and communicate with spirits. Many rainforest shamans simply refer to Ayahuasca as 'el remedio,' the remedy."

He goes on to say, "Ayahuasca was never used casually or for recreational purposes in traditional societies. Only a ritually clean person who maintained a strict dietary regimen (low on spices, sugars and animal fat) for several weeks or months was deemed ready to partake of the experience. Shamanic initiation rites entailed a lengthy period of preparation, which included social isolation and sexual abstinence (requirements Jerry does not feel are necessary) before novices got to ingest yage (Ayahuasca)."

Ayahuasca, also referred by some as "yage", can have dreadful side effects, according to Lee. He says after the brew is ingested, "A vertiginous surge of energy envelops them (the participants). And then all hell breaks loose: retching, vomiting, diarrhea—an unstoppable high colonic that penetrates the innards, sweeping through the intestinal coils like liquid Drano of the soul, cleansing the body of parasites, emotional blockages, long-held resentments. It is for good reason the Amazonian natives refer to 'la purga' when speaking of yage."

Lee quotes Sonoma-based psychologist Ralph Metzner, editor of "Ayahuasca, an anthology of scholarly and first person accounts of the yage experience." He notes that there have been "anecdotal reports of the complete remission of some cancers after one or two Ayahuasca sessions. The rejuvenating impact of la purga would help explain the exceptional health of the ayahuasqueros (Shamen who use the concoction in their ceremonies), even those of advanced age."

There are also a number of uncredited writings on the Internet concerning Ayahuasca: "It is remarkable and significant that at least seventy-two different indigenous tribes of Amazonia, however widely separated by long distance, language and cultural differences, all manifested a detailed common knowledge of Ayahuasca and its uses."

Back in his class, Jerry continued to explain that a liver-cleanse would help mitigate the side effects. He recommends a book, <u>The Amazing Liver and Gallbladder Cleanse</u> by Andreas Moritz (www.Ener-Chi.com), and promises to supply all-natural remedies to any who are interested.

They then moved on to "seeing energy." Jerry used a small crystal he said will help his students see energy waves coming off their fingertips. Jerry called it a Guardian crystal. "It's made of solid gold," he said. "It was developed as a result of a dream."

Jerry went on to tell them how it worked. "There are a couple of batteries in here. There's the crystal. There is the gold. There is the light. There is no bulb in this."

Jerry turned the cap attached to the crystal and it lit up. The crystal, about an inch long, glowed faintly red.

In pairs, Jerry's students took the crystal into a dark room, and held it up to their fingers. "Immediately you will see a glow like a fog around your fingers," Jerry said. "The more you look, the more detail you will see. The detail you are looking for: tiny, tiny hair like fingers of energy coming off the crystal, almost a curling effect. If you get your focus right and start looking you may even see little spots of light just exploding in the air like little balls of light that just sort of pop into place."

Jerry explained that healing is all about seeing energy. "When I work with a person to see what is going on inside of them," Jerry said, "the first thing I do is look at their field. That's the glowing essence you see around the crystal. That's the field."

One of the students asked what happens to that energy when you die.

"When a person dies," Jerry answered, "there is a flash of light almost like a flash bulb goes off. The essence that was there is gone. It just doesn't look the same. A piece of wood has a very similar glow to it. It was something that was once living, once vital."

The class discussion turned to using energy to heal, how to manipulate it, how to generate it in your hands to use it on someone.

"For me it's a natural gift or an instinct," Jerry said. "But for a person who is wanting to develop it, it's basically a point of perspective, and a degree of knowledge. I believe that with the right perspective and the right amount of knowledge, you can have the experience. Knowing how to use it is going to be something that is wisdom-oriented. But wisdom comes with time and experience."

By the end of the session, everyone in the class said they could see energy from the crystal. Some said they could see it on Jerry's hands, and their own hands. Progress was being made.

For homework, Jerry wanted them to practice seeing energy. He also wanted them to practice on a plant. "Start using the plant to focus energy on the leaves, around the plant and around the soil. When you give the plant some water, hold the water and put some energy into it. Then give it to the plant to drink."

He also reminded his students to consider a liver cleanse.

In the next session, Jerry and his students worked with sound. They went over Jerry's map of energy points on the body, and discussed how energy flows through the body, and where it can be measured.

He also passed out two typed sheets of paper for their healer "toolbox." One was something Jerry called the "Healer's Prayer." The other was his "Healer's Mantra."

Jerry read the Healer's Prayer to his students:

> Connect me to the universe
> The mind of God
> Connect me to compassion
> The heart of God
> Connect me to the Earth
> The Manifested Garden of God
> Connect me to Infinity
> The Realm of God
> Connect me to Others
> The Image of God

> Connect me that I represent the
Greatest Good
>> I connect to the flow of creation
>> And embrace the will of God.

"I know each of you have your own prayer that you use," Jerry said. "And I'm not suggesting that this should take the place of anything you are already using. But consider it as another tool."

Jerry told the class how he originally received the prayer. "I always enjoyed listening to the wind as I rode my BMW touring bike," he said. "I wish I still had one! Though it might sound crazy, I could hear music and conversations as the wind rushed past my ears. The melodies or spoken words were easy to hear since I never wore a helmet. About six years ago, as Kathy and I drove to the east coast, the air conditioner broke down in our old Suburban. We were crossing southern Colorado. It was pretty warm, and we had the windows opened. Quite hot and uncomfortable, I decided to lean my head against the opened window frame to hear the rush of the wind. Within a few minutes I started hearing familiar music in the wind. Then, something unexpected happened. I heard a voice so clear it startled me. As I listened, a mysterious voice recited the same phrase several times. After finishing, it began again. The voice was powerful and compelling. I wondered what I was listening to. The voice told me this was a prayer I could use before I started working with someone in need. Within minutes I found our trip notebook and wrote down what I had heard. I still listen to the wind…I guess that's why I enjoy sitting near waterfalls or atop mountain peaks in the Andes."

Jerry then told the students about his Healer's Mantra. "It is actually something that occurred to me one night, in an instant," he said. "And because Kathy suggested I get up immediately and write it down, I have it still today."

Jerry told his class that he didn't realize at the time he was writing it down that it was as powerful a tool as it ended up being. "And the way this is powerful," Jerry told them, "probably is best explained first." He went on to explain the power of the spoken word.

Jerry gave them an example. "Simply saying 'I am at peace,' and meditating on that for a moment brings about dramatic changes within your spiritual and energetic body. I suggest you take each line, or couple of lines if the entire phrase requires it, and meditate on this - recite it to yourself several times as you breathe deeply between recitations. Whether each line is spoken singularly or the entire composition spoken at once, the Healer's Mantra has a beautiful effect on your state of being. Regardless of how you personally choose to read this, please take a slow breath between each line and let the intention and inspiration of each passage expand within you."

He then read them the Healer's Mantra:

I Am Peace
I Am Love
I Am Eternity
I Am But One Image of God
Perfect & Whole
I Am Responsible for His Garden
I Am Co-Creator of the Universe
Never Separated
Always Connected
Before My Next Step I Have Created the
Firmament
Before My Next Breath I Create the
Atmosphere
As I Open My Eyes I Create All I Will
See
My Face Is God's Mirror
The Light From My Eyes Is Creation's
Radiance
I Am Complete Peace, Love and Eternity
I Am, And Have Always Been, Eternal
I Am But One Image of God, Perfect and
Whole
My Soul Is Not Just Within, But
Surrounds Me and All Whom I Encounter
I Am The Spirit and Essence of The Earth
I Am The Cosmos
I Am The Image Of God Finally
Revealed
Look Deep Within Me to See Yourself
As I See You

> See Yourself As I Have Seen Myself
> You Are But One Image Of God
> Perfect and Whole
> Our Existence Provides Us A Simple, Yet
> Powerful Truth
> God Lives Here…

Jerry said, "I figured this would be another nice tool for you to use. And if you use this tool over and over and over again, I believe that it will be as empowering for you as it has been for me."

They then went on to talk more about healing, and the spoken word. In a dramatic demonstration, Jerry showed them how to shout "mantras." One student would stand next to another and shout whatever came to mind or whatever they thought would have a positive impact on the "client's" energy field. Many of the students said they could feel a powerful burst of energy as the mantras were shouted at them.

At one point, Jerry played "Wayanakuy," a beautiful and haunting song recorded by Alborada, a group of shamen from South America. After the song was played, Jerry told them, "I don't know what they are saying. It just sounds good. It's melodic, it's rhythmic, and it sounds good. Everything that runs in the body is melodic and rhythmic, and when you start putting this kind of sound and emotional force to work, using your own voice, you start compelling things outside of you as well as inside of you."

312

The class practiced more with sound and melodic rhythm. One of the students thought that just saying the word "God" had an impact on him.

"That's exactly in line with what I am trying to convey to you guys," Jerry replied. "It doesn't really matter what you say as long as what you say means something to you."

In their next gathering, Jerry got down to more practical matters of being a healer. They talked about legal guidelines. Jerry recommended a book titled <u>Legal Guidelines for Unlicensed Practitioners</u>. Jerry discovered long ago that it was necessary to take certain legal precautions when doing work as a healer.

They also talked about how to analyze a person's health issues. "We legally cannot and should never use the word diagnosis," Jerry said. "A diagnosis is an action that belongs to someone else."

Jerry told them the book has a list of words that shouldn't be used by someone not licensed to practice medicine. Using those words could open them up to criminal or civil actions.

One of the students asked Jerry about using the term "cancer."

Jerry gave them an example. "A client described her condition to me, as told to her by her physician, that she had cancer. I agreed that I saw something that might be called cancer in her, and that I was going to do my best to eliminate it. I unconsciously used the word cancer. I should have been more aware and not done this. But like the woman I was working on, I became emotionally connected and spoke with her as any friend would. I was concerned for her emotional state of being because she had been told it was very likely she was going to die soon. I didn't follow the instructions I've given you today and placed myself at an unnecessary risk. It's important to think before you speak. Understand that regardless what your perception is of the issue you encounter, you cannot use certain terms or phrases. Furthermore, you could be mistaken and add to their anxiety unnecessarily. Always practice awareness and you will be fine."

Jerry said they have to use their own judgment. "There are those who might want to stop you from helping others, no matter how effective you are. You have to consider this and become very clear that entrapment is a risk. There are people that would come in and say, 'I've got a bad arthritic shoulder here. Man, this hurts so bad! Do you see any arthritis there?' They want to trick you into saying, 'Oh, look at all that arthritis you have.' Then it will be, 'Ha! I got you. Turn around and face the wall!' I'm not teaching you this to make you afraid. I'm relating this to help you avoid a frightening event that is completely unnecessary."

Jerry also discussed working with node points, giving his students more insight on how to detect the pathways and important energy distribution points within the human energy flow.

314

The sixth and final class took place in Peru. Most of the students went there with Jerry about a month later. Some did not. Those who traveled to Peru spent time with both an Amazon rainforest and Andean mountain shaman; they drank Ayahuasca and participated in ancient rites of passage and rituals. "My students journeyed deep into mystical realms," Jerry said. "That few from our culture have ever had a chance to experience."

For Jerry, taking a group like his class to Peru has always been special. "Each who have traveled this path before you have stood at the boundary between life and death, and wondered what is just beyond," Jerry wrote on his website. "Their journey into what seemed as death was only a step into and through a multidimensional, multifaceted universe where the only barriers that exist are within the minds of those whose dreams and imaginations are limited."

Chapter Fourteen
True Believer

Viola Johnson (everyone calls her Vi) is a fifty-four-year-old registered nurse who lives in Aberdeen, Maryland. She works at the Spring Grove Hospital Center in Catonsville, a medical care facility that has taken care of people since the 1700's.

Viola has been a nurse for thirty years, and married for thirty-four.

She's had all kinds of health problems, not the least of which was arthritis. Viola had a hard time getting around and wasn't finding much help. She also had severe breathing problems – most likely asthma caused by dust or pollen, or other pollutants in the atmosphere.

A spiritual person, one day Viola asked for divine intervention. "When I had these physical problems," Viola said, "I was praying for God's will because I was in such a bad state that all I wanted was God's will and God's way."

She said it was one coincidence after another that led her to Jerry Wills. "All of a sudden, something said look up South America on the computer," she said. "I couldn't imagine why it said South America, and then it said click on the Amazon. I thought how is this going to help? Then it said look up shamanism, and I thought this is ridiculous. But I clicked on shamanism and from there I was led to a medical intuitive, and from there I was led to Jerry. It was an amazing series of coincidences."

She said it was more than just a feeling that led her to Jerry. "It was a real consciousness thing, knowing that I was being led. It was a strong feeling because I wanted to click on the best hospitals…you know something like that. But instead, something was leading me to Peru, leading me to Jerry."

Viola didn't know Jerry at the time. But after seeing his website and reading more about shamanism, she decided to give him a call. "I stopped analyzing and stopped questioning and just did what my intuitive skills led me to do."

Jerry told her he could do a long distance healing session, by phone. He said healers like him don't necessarily have to be in the same room as their client. Long distance healing was a skill Jerry had developed over the years, and was now confident enough to try it on people like Viola.

"I talked to Jerry about my sensitivity to toxins in the environment," Viola said. "I told him it had gotten so bad I was almost afraid to breathe."

Jerry told her she'd never be afraid to breathe again. "So he worked on that at first," she said. "He did whatever it is that he does, and since then I've never had any problems with breathing, I haven't had a reaction of any kind."

Viola said she didn't have to fear not being able to breathe. "All of a sudden I was clear, I could breathe, and I went into areas that I was previously not able to breathe in, and it was still clear."

Viola's arthritis was next. "I went down steps one at a time," she said. "And I had just finished a rehabilitation evaluation, and I was declared handicapped." Viola's circulation was poor as well. Her ankles would often turn blue. She was also overweight, which didn't help much. "I had to use one arm of the chair to push up with. I couldn't stand normally out of a seat. I had to sit in a chair with arms on it so I could get up."

She also had a very persistent and noticeable limp in her right leg. "My right leg was bent. It would not straighten. Now one leg was longer than the other. Not because it started out that way, but because it was bent when I walked; it made one leg shorter than the other," she said.

She also had constant pain in almost every joint. About all her doctors did for her was provide arthritis medication.

As a nurse, she was on her feet almost all day. "In order to be on my feet all day long and keep up with the rest of the staff, I would have to dose up on my pain meds and arthritis meds just to keep up," she said. "Just to be able to stand. There was nothing else left for me except a wheel chair."

For her arthritis, Jerry did a series of healings over the phone. He also recommended vitamins and natural foods to help Viola with her weight problem. "I did a liver cleanse three times.

I just did what Jerry recommended." Nine months later, Viola had lost a hundred pounds. "And I had much better mental clarity," she said.

The pain in her joints went away. "I really couldn't believe it," she said. "People could not believe the difference in me. I had no pain in my shoulders. I had really swollen finger joints; the swelling in my finger joints went down completely."

And Viola was off pain medication.

She strongly believes the long distance healing worked. "When Jerry worked on me, I could feel my joints loosening. I could actually feel them moving while we were on the phone," she said. "If, for example, I complained to him about neck pain, he would work on it, and it was gone."

Before seeing Jerry, it was hard for her to just get up in the morning. "I would wake up in the morning, and I would not be able to walk. I would have to sit there for a while to get myself together. Now I just jumped up out of bed."

During one of her healing sessions, Jerry told Viola she would be going with him to Peru someday soon. "I thought to myself, oh, you're dreaming," Viola said. "I didn't even believe it, so I talked to him about something else, but then he said again, 'You are going to Peru, and we're going to have a great time.' Again, I thought, oh yeah, there was just no way I could get there."

But believe it or not, Viola continued to progress and continued to lose weight. Within a few months, even she was ready to go with Jerry to Peru. "I decided to go," she said, "to have more of what we call a consciousness expansion, to become more consciously aware of energy as a result of being exposed to energy there. I signed up for the trip. I went by myself."

One of the first things Viola did was tell everyone on the tour about Jerry. "I told other people about my right leg, which had straightened out." But even while on the tour, Viola had some problems. "I was still going up steps one at a time."

She also credits more work with Jerry, and her trip to Peru. "Being exposed to all that energy in Peru helped me," she said. "There are places in Peru that are associated with natural energy, so that along with Jerry's work - that sort of enabled me to just do some phenomenal things that otherwise I never would have been able to do."

The best example came when Jerry took his tour group up to Marcahuasi – a 13,000 foot plateau in Peru.

After the bus ride to San Pedro de Casta, Viola wasn't sure she could make the trip up to the top by horseback. So she decided to stay behind.

Jerry made sure Viola had accommodations in town, then led the horse ride up the side of the mountain to Marcahuasi.

Just imagine his surprise when the very next morning he saw Viola standing there. He had just gotten up, and there she was standing there at the top of the hill.

Jerry said, "How did you get up here?"

"I walked," she said.

Jerry stood there amazed. He and everyone in the group wondered how in the world Viola accomplished such a feat.

"I've walked seven miles since five o'clock this morning and climbed three thousand feet, almost straight up," Viola said later. "It was a climb over rough terrain, too."

It wasn't just a sudden improvement in her physical skills that Viola noticed. "When I got up there," she said, "my intuitive skills became more clear, more sharpened. I was in my tent that one night, and I woke up like two or three in the morning when you are half awake, and half asleep, and I looked at the side of my tent and it wasn't there. I could see the mountain right through my tent."

Viola said it was all about being exposed to the energy in Peru. "As a result of being exposed to this energy, you have more vibration energy within your body. You gain more intuitive skills. Your perceptions become increased, and you begin to see energy." Viola said she also gained a special skill. "I can see energy. Energy is alive all around us."

She also said her ability to get around improved dramatically while in Peru. "My leg became completely straight," she said. "I had no stiffness. I walked for seven hours straight, and you are talking to someone who could barely walk across the room."

Viola's self-confidence had grown by leaps and bounds. "I am a person who prays," she said, "and I've had some miraculous things that happened to me physically as a result of prayer."

For Viola, the healing sessions with Jerry and the physical improvement and mental clarity she gained in Peru were all part of a plan – one just for her. "You have these experiences and coincidences in your life that just start unfolding that cue you into the fact that something else is happening. You can call it evolution because you are evolving as a person. Your consciousness is evolving, so you have higher thoughts. You get in touch with more wisdom; you start to get rid of the anger you might have felt. Your energy collapses when you are angry or fearful. You learn to control those negative emotions. You get a lot more positive, and you get a lot more connected with people."

Clearly, Viola is a true believer, especially after what has happened to her. She tries to convince other people to give Jerry a try as well. "I try to impress people with the fact that it is real," she said. "One person said to me the other day, 'Well, that must be psychological.' So I think if you don't see it for yourself, it's like the person doesn't understand it. It has to be put to a person in a way where they think, well, maybe you are right. And then when they say, 'Well, maybe.' It leads them to the next step."

For Jerry, Viola has been a wonderful success story. But like many people he works on, there was no instant gratification. It doesn't always work right away. It took several sessions with Viola to get her problems under control. He also needed her cooperation when it came to weight loss. Without Viola's determination to stick to her cleansing, diet, and positive attitude, Jerry most likely would have had a much more difficult time turning her around.

"It disturbs me a little when I work on someone, and there isn't just an instantaneous flash of wellness that takes over," Jerry said. "It doesn't always happen that way." Jerry said it's one of the big joys he gets out of life when results are instantaneous. "I like to see the results of a miracle first hand. It's fun. It's a joy."

Jerry often says that his healings don't always work, and there are different reasons why. "If they (his clients) completely accept where they are, and they're not willing to accept things differently, then it's very difficult to convince their minds that something has happened." For some people, Jerry says, their sickness or injury has become too big a part of who they are. "Because they completely accept where they are. Some people even receive love this way, and some people give love this way, by being sick."

Sometimes it's just too late to do any good.

Several years ago, Jerry was called to work on a man we will call James (Not his real name).

The man had been a professional journalist and photographer his entire adult life. His work had gained him worldwide fame for more than fifty years, and his personal photographic achievements occurred during some of the most tumultuous years in American history. His pictures still are used in history books, newspapers and magazines the world over.

Jerry first met James in the spring by his bedside in the hospital. James had been suffering from heart problems which had become more serious. And just hours before Jerry met him, James had suffered a stroke. Now barely coherent, James could not speak. His face was paralyzed and drawn on one side. Jerry knew the situation was not good.

Jerry had been called by a close friend to help James. And as usual, Jerry hated the hospital surroundings he found himself in. The feeling of sickness and desperation haunted the halls like a bad smell Jerry could never completely identify with, or move away from. Patients and their families wandered from rooms to waiting areas and back again, heads bowed and tired of the events forcing them to be there. Jerry had become so familiar with the sights and smells associated with hospitals, that it took a great deal of strength just to be there.

Jerry walked up to James' bed and sat in a small chair beside him. As a friend closed the door, separating Jerry from the busy nurses attending their patients and ringing phone calls, Jerry closed his eyes and began to focus. Within a few minutes he felt the silent rush of energy flowing through his body. He could no longer hear the respirator or IV machines pumping. Heat spread into his hands as the energy flowed towards them.

Opening his eyes, Jerry looked towards James as he lay there. Jerry carefully lifted his hand and held it between both of his. "Images immediately filled my mind's eye," Jerry said. "I immediately witnessed aspects of his life play out in rapid motion. Finally the images subsided, and now I was looking at his condition."

As Jerry's attention moved through James' body, he saw his damaged heart. "From there I moved upwards toward his neck and finally his head," Jerry said. "His condition was serious."

Always following his first inclinations, Jerry's experience taught him to direct his attention to where the most serious problems were.

Gently placing his hands on James' head, Jerry directed energy towards the several small blood clots peppering his brain. One by one, the tiny clots dissolved. As Jerry gazed deeper into James' brain, he could see another larger clot near the center left hemisphere. As Jerry manifested and focused more energy on the larger clot, it too started to dissolve away.

As usual, the energy stopped when Jerry finished his work. He felt the heat leave his hands, and his awareness was no longer engaged in a manner allowing him to see inside James. Instead, Jerry was left with a feeling of completion.

"James slowly opened his eyes and looked at me," Jerry said. "Still unable to speak, he seemed more at peace and more alert than when I first entered the room."

A few minutes later, Jerry was in his car headed home. James' improving condition had impressed everyone. By the end of the week, James was well enough to be moved to a nearby private nursing facility.

But the success Jerry had treating James was short lived. James had continued to improve until one morning he suffered another stroke. Jerry was asked to help once again.

James was unconscious when Jerry arrived.

As Jerry prepared himself to work on James once more, he suddenly saw an image of the man standing beside his own bed. "James pointed to his body on the bed," Jerry said. "And he said, 'I can't breathe.'"

Jerry walked over to the bed and saw that James' breathing tube, which was obscured by other medical equipment, was clogged. It was filled with phlegm. Jerry immediately called the nurse. "He can't breathe. His breathing tube is full of phlegm and yucky stuff," Jerry told her.

The nurse checked the tube, and said, "How did you know?"

Jerry said he had talked to the man. He had an out of body experience and told Jerry he couldn't breathe.

"Oh my God," said the nurse. "I've seen you before. You were on FOX TV! You are the guy who works on sick people. You worked on that man in Chandler!"

Jerry realized she must have seen the story on FOX-10 News. "Yes, that was me," he said.

"Oh, God bless you," the nurse said. "You're here to help him." Then she called some orderlies to help her clean the breathing tube.

The breathing issue resolved, Jerry again saw the man out of body. This time he told Jerry he was waiting for his son to come see him. He'd had a falling out with his son. But the family had already told Jerry that his son wasn't coming to see him.

"Looking fresh and vibrant as he appeared to me again, he spoke in a soft tone of how grateful he was I had come to help him," Jerry said as he later described the encounter. "He told me he had made a decision and asked me to stop assisting him. James appreciated all I had done to help and now had one final request."

Jerry was asked to relay a message to James' mother and daughter. "James explained how he had been rejected by his son in the last few years because he had spent so much time traveling as a journalist. He explained that he had wanted to live long enough to reconcile with his son. If only he

328

had another chance to say how sorry he was for his parental failures and lack of loving attention."

James' heart attack and subsequent stroke had prevented him from reconciling with his son. And he told Jerry he was relieved that his help had offered him another chance.

Though his daughter had come to see him, James' son still refused. "It was now sadly obvious to him that his son would not come," Jerry said.

As James looked toward his still body, he now told Jerry how tired he was. "He had had a rewarding life," Jerry said. "Life as an invalid was not for him. He knew he would never recover and did not want to live."

Jerry looked towards James and nodded yes. "I told him the choice had always been his to make," Jerry said. "James told me his time was finished, and though a little concerned, he was looking forward to whatever came next. I told him to simply relax and seek the essence of God within." Jerry also told him to follow his feelings.

Again, James thanked Jerry and then seemed to simply fade from Jerry's view.

Slowly, Jerry regained his composure as he stood and walked toward the hospital waiting area. James' daughter and elderly mother were still waiting patiently. Jerry relayed the message James had given him about his son.

Finally, Jerry told them that James wanted to leave. "Though they did not want to accept this, it was clear they knew his time was near," Jerry said.

"They promised each other to sit with James around the clock, confident that should he once again awaken he would find them there. James would not die alone."

James never regained consciousness and died a few hours later with both family members sitting beside him, holding his hands. "I felt privileged to have met him," Jerry said. Helping James pass on was an example of how Jerry could still help someone, even if he couldn't heal.

"There is little we can do when it's our time to go," Jerry explained. "But the human spirit can hold on long enough to help those around us prepare if the need is great enough. In James' instance, it was clear he wanted time to allow his son an opportunity to make things right between them. James had already forgiven his son for the alienation. He understood his death would prevent the two of them from reconciling the feelings of abandonment his son had for such a long time. I believe James wanted to spare his son from the eventual sadness of having lost the chance to reconcile with his father. James allowed me to assist only to the point he felt comfortable holding on. When he realized his son was not coming, he decided to go.

A similar incident happened to Jerry sometime later in Peoria, Arizona. "This woman had cancer, and the family asked me to come over and help her," Jerry said. "I went to help her, and she was like, 'There are dogs on fire!' She had lost her mind and was hallucinating. I walked up to help her and she went completely lucid right away. She said, 'No, don't.' So I backed off, and she went all wacky again."

In this case, Jerry could only help the family prepare for the woman's death. "There was nothing I could do to help her. She actually told me not to."

Jerry said there have been other times when he's worked with people, and nothing happens. "It turns out that what I was there to do wasn't really to do the obvious thing. And it's different with every circumstance, but I think I'm there to help them be better, and sometimes I'm not there for that reason. I'm there for something else, and I don't even know what it is sometimes."

Jerry can usually tell right away when it is someone's time to go, but not always. "Because I may be emotionally connected to them, or I may be too emotionally connected to the outcome, or because I don't want someone to pass away."

Sometimes, Jerry doesn't know until he touches the person he is trying to save. "Most of the time, if I tap into a person and it's not going to work, my hands go icy cold. And no matter what, I can't pull my energy level up, not even to a normal level. My energy level drops down below normal, and I can feel that. As soon as I pull away from a person, my energy level comes back up."

"I think it must be God's will, or the will of whatever is involved here," Jerry continued.

"Because when it's their time, there's no changing that. And I'm not allowed to interfere with it. If I really pushed the issue, I think I probably could. But I don't know what the repercussions would be from doing something like that. I haven't gotten up the courage to give it a try."

There are those clients who come to see Jerry for treatment of a non-life threatening ailment. And when nothing happens in these cases, they want to know why. "You didn't do anything," they say.

"I did do something," counters Jerry. "I showed up and God was here, but this was in your path. This is part of your experience, and I can't interfere."

Jerry said he's not going to take it upon himself to feel bad or guilty when nothing happens. He tells his disappointed clients, "This is part of God's plan. It's not part of mine. You know, if it were my will that was involved, I would have a great time with this. The children's hospital would be my first stop."

Chapter Fifteen
Laying on of Hands

Taking a break from the experiences and knowledge of Jerry Wills, in this chapter we're going to take a closer look at energy healing, or as some call it, the "Laying on of Hands."

The laying on of hands is "a religious practice found throughout the world in varying forms," according to the free on-line encyclopedia Wikipedia (Which anyone can contribute to). It goes on to say, "In Christian churches, this practice is used as both a symbolic and formal method of invoking the Holy Spirit during baptisms, healing services and ordination of priests, ministers, elders, deacons and other church officers."

Other sources, including the Bible, are filled with ceremony and healing involving the laying on of hands. In Matthew 8:14-15 RSV, "And when Jesus entered Peter's house, He saw his mother-in-law lying sick with a fever; He touched her hand, and the fever left her, and she rose and served Him."

In Luke 22:50-51 RSV, "And one of them struck the slave of the high priest and cut off his right ear. But Jesus said, "No more of this!" And He touched his ear and healed him."

In modern times, the laying on of hands is an act followed by many religions. In his paper on

Baptists practices, Walter B. Shurden, the executive director for the Center of Baptist Studies writes, "Today Baptists usually associate laying on hands with the ordination of deacons or clergy. However, Baptists possess another tradition of laying on hands that is deeply rooted in their history. I refer, of course, to the laying on of hands on believers following their baptism. It is a remarkable symbol where new Christians received through the church the blessing of Almighty God."

There is no doubt that the laying on of hands was a means of connecting the message with the messenger, especially in the early church. Throughout history it provided a way of authenticating some sort of spiritual gift or message. Jesus is often quoted by historians or theologians as saying the laying on of hands would be involved in the gift of healing as his followers went about ministering the gift of healing.

But when it comes to laying on of hands beyond the days that Jesus walked the Earth, the church of today finds little in common with the practice and healing. Now the laying on of hands is mostly confined to the formal ceremony by which the church commissions those selected into their formal service…including ordainment or baptism.

In today's world, the laying on of hands by anyone not ordained by a known church or other established religious practice is usually called faith healing or energy healing. And it is either something you practice and believe in – or something considered common fraud.

Those who claim fraud runs rampant in the energy healing community point to what they consider a truly comprehensive examination of healers: James Randi's book, <u>The Faith Healers</u>. In his book, Randi, a celebrated magician, and his team of researchers attended several healing services, and were pronounced healed of the fake diseases they claimed to have. According to an internet ad for Randi's book, "The ministries, they (Randi's researchers) discovered, were rife with deception, chicanery, and often outright fraud."

What Randi writes is really nothing new. There is little doubt that fraud is common in many traveling or televangelical ministries. Many have been exposed on national newscasts or well known periodicals.

One of Randi's most spectacular cases involved Peter Popoff, whom the magician exposed on "The Johnny Carson Show." Popoff became famous for calling out the names of people in his audience and then describing their ailments. Popoff said he received his information from God. But he was disgraced when investigators recorded Popoff's wife reading information over a wireless communication system to her husband, information surreptitiously obtained by associates who mingled with the crowd before each performance. Popoff could hear what his wife was saying by wearing a hidden earpiece. (By the way, after his national disgrace, Popoff is back. You can catch his act still on some televangelical broadcasts across the country.)

Besides those who write books and appear on talk shows exposing bogus healers, there are others who take a more scientific approach to discrediting the healing community. Dr. Barry L. Beyerstein, PhD. writes on the website, www.quackwatch.com that there are often scientific explanations for why a healer appears to succeed in his mission to heal. Beyerstein writes:

> "There are at least seven reasons why people may erroneously conclude that an ineffective therapy works: 1. The disease may have run its natural course... 2. Many diseases are cyclical. Such conditions as arthritis, multiple sclerosis, allergies and gastrointestinal problems normally have ups and downs... 3. The placebo effect may be responsible. Through suggestion, belief, expectancy, cognitive reinterpretation, and diversion of attention, patients given biologically useless treatments often experience measurable relief.... 4. People who hedge their bets credit the wrong thing. If improvement occurs after someone has had both "alternative" and science-based treatment, the fringe practice often gets a disproportionate share of the credit. 5. The original diagnosis or prognosis may have

been incorrect… 6. Temporary mood improvement can be confused with a cure… 7. Psychological needs can distort what people perceive and do. Even when no objective improvement occurs, people with a strong psychological investment in "alternative medicine" can convince themselves they have been helped."

Dr. Beyerstein makes some interesting points – especially when you consider how many patients get traditional treatments along with non-traditional energy healing. It's sometimes difficult to separate the two.

His point on psychological needs is also similar to arguments made by other skeptics who claim faith healing is nothing more than a form of hypnosis. According to this theory, the so-called healers only convince their "patients" that they are feeling better…that what healers do is nothing more than some form of mind control.

But what few people have been exposed to is some of the work being done now to measure energy healing quantitatively in a controlled scientific environment.

Dr. Melinda Connor has been conducting a study of energy healers and energy healing in Tucson, Arizona. Dr. Connor is the Director of the Karen Connor Optimal Healing Research program at the Laboratory for Advances in Consciousness and Health (LACH for short) at the University of

Arizona. She holds an MA in Counseling Psychology from the University of San Francisco and a Ph.D. in Clinical Psychology from California Coast University. And her current research focuses on Biofield therapies.

Dr. Connor works alongside Dr. Gary Schwartz, who runs all the research at LACH. Gary Schwartz, Ph.D., is a professor of Psychology, Medicine, Neurology, Psychiatry, and Surgery at the University of Arizona. He is also the Director of The VERITAS Research Program of the Human Energy Systems Laboratory in the Department of Psychology at the University of Arizona. He received his Ph.D. from Harvard University. Dr. Schwartz is the co-author of The Living Energy Universe, and is the author of The Truth About Medium and The Afterlife Experiments: Breakthrough Scientific Evidence of Life After Death. He's also recently published The Healing Experiments, using much of the data Dr. Connor and others gathered. Dr. Schwartz has also published several hundred scientific papers and edited still several other academic books.

Dr. Schwartz's major research focus has been in the controversial field of parapsychology-- which has exposed him to all kinds of ridicule, especially from those people who haven't taken the time to read his books or examine the data collected at his lab. The so-called super-skeptics (Like Randi) of anything and everything paranormal have singled him out for special ridicule. It's been both unfair and inaccurate because rarely if ever are his actual findings discussed.

The Laboratory for Advances in Consciousness and Health, according to Schwartz, integrates mind-body medicine, energy medicine and spiritual medicine.

When people ask Schwartz what he does in the lab, he says he works in what may be considered three controversial areas. "One is controversial," he said. "The second is very controversial. The third is super-controversial."

The just controversial area involves mind medicine. "We focus in the areas of meditation healing on long term health," Schwartz said. "Not terribly controversial.

"The very controversial," Schwartz continued, "is in the area of energy medicine. We take a look at bioelectric magnetic recordings or different signals from the body, including magnetism and electric cardiograms going out into space. This may relate to things like therapeutic touch."

The super-controversial gets really interesting. "The super-controversial," he explained, "is in the area of spiritual medicine and spiritual systems science. What that means in plain English is the possibility of survival of consciousness after death, and what we call the SAM hypothesis for Spirit Assisted Medicine."

Schwartz was no true believer in this stuff; at least he didn't start out that way. "I started out very skeptical," he said. "I was raised an orthodox agnostic, which is exactly how I approach things, questioning but open minded." Schwartz said he is not cynical. "But I'm from Missouri; you have to show me. And you have to show me again and show me again before I finally believe."

No matter what your subject, be it rocket science or energy healing, Dr. Schwartz said he believed in the fundamental principles of science. "Like the science of healing," he said, "is to make observations and to describe those observations. Then determine if they are replicable observations. That is the number one basis of science. Science is not a set of theories about what is true and not true. It's not about what is believable or not believable, what is possible or not possible. Science is about a methodology of studying nature, studying the world around us."

Schwartz said it is all about keeping open minds. "Science is not supposed to be only self correcting, but it is also supposed to be self evolving. We are supposed to be able to change our minds as a function of the new data that comes in."

Accusations of "pseudo-science" are often leveled against Schwartz and his colleagues. But most who make the accusations have never actually read the data the lab has collected over the years. In The Afterlife Experiments, Dr. Schwartz and his colleagues put to the test some of the country's best known mediums – those who can communicate with the dead. They included John Edward, Suzane

Northrop and George Anderson. He wrote a separate book, <u>The Truth About Medium</u>, about experiments conducted with the real Allison DuBois of the NBC-TV drama "Medium."

I'm not going into many details here. If you want more, read his books. I have, and the data is startling. Dr. Schwartz and his team conducted blind and double-blind experiments. The mediums did not know whom they were talking to or for whom they were providing information. The experiments were also done in a controlled laboratory environment. There was no way for the mediums to cheat. And the results were impressive. Many had accuracy rates as high as 90%.

"There was a great line by a man named Sir William Crookes," Schwartz said. "Which goes something like, 'I did not say it was possible, I said it happened.' Isn't that a great line? For me, I reframe it slightly. I say, 'If it happens, it is possible.'"

For more on the energy healing experiments being conducted at the lab, Dr. Schwartz recommended I talk to Dr. Melinda Connor. He calls her "The Michael Jordan" of energy healers. She also ran the lab's experiments on human energy fields.

A few months later, I met with Dr. Connor at the lab. The facility is housed off-campus as part of what appears to be a common medical mall made up of small one-story beige buildings set around a large parking lot in north-central Tucson.

Doctor Connor greeted me at the door, and in her very friendly manner, offered to show me around the laboratory.

We walked through several small rooms at the lab. Each one housed equipment for different experiments. In one room, there was a device that measured gamma and x-rays from healers when they were "running energy." Connor used the term "running energy" like other healers who use it to describe the state of being they enter when a healing session begins. For example, when Jerry Wills begins to focus for a healing session, and looks inside a person to see what is wrong, he would be "running energy" in Connor's use of the phrase. Dr. Connor said her early data showed changes in x-ray and gamma-ray fields when the healers who are being tested "run energy."

In another room, Connor described the machine inside as a laser profusion imager. She said, "We're in the process of looking at capillary dilation changes and heat."

In other words, they want to know why a healer's hands suddenly become hot when running energy. "We are testing to see whether or not the oscillatory effect that we get isn't also a factor in micro-movement of the capillary system and micro-movement of the muscle system."

Connor believes something is happening to the natural body rhythms of the healer when they run energy. They're not sure what or why, but the changes do occur, and increased blood flow to capillaries in the hands may be a part of it.

As she explains it, "The body breathes. You inhale and you exhale. That is an oscillatory process. Your heart beats-- that is an oscillatory process. You put your foot down; that is a percussion oscillatory process. It shakes the body as you put the foot down." She says healers were producing a change in their baseline oscillatory rate that they can measure. "It (the oscillatory rate) is different when the healer is just sitting and talking about doing their grocery shopping, versus when they are actually running energy.

"It appears healers are doing something physical, that it's not just intention. Intention is not manifestation. There's a process of movement from intention into manifestation that is taking place. What we saw was a change in (the healer's) oscillatory rate. And it was a very, very dramatic one. There is a physical change in their body."

In another room, researchers do bio-photon imaging of healers working on plant leaves. Connor said the results of tests in this room dramatically showed the effects healers could have on a plant leaf.

When Connor and her colleagues ran experiments in this room, they placed a white piece of paper on the top of two identical tables--the only furniture in the room. On top of each sheet of identical paper they placed two mature leafs pulled from the same plant. Above each table was a desk lamp; both lamps were the exact same kind, with the exact same light bulb. The two lamps shone brightly on each leaf as all other lights in the room were turned off. The distance between the lamps and the two leaves were identical. The temperature was also controlled and steady. A healer then entered the room and sat at one of the desks (and as the experiments were run repeatedly with the same healer or different healer, they would switch desks). Without touching the leaf in any way, the healer then ran energy to the leaf, actually stimulating it to release energy faster and glow brighter.

Remember when Jerry Wills was pulling weeds from the garden in his front yard? He saw light coming from the wounded weed stems and leaves. According to Connor, this is what happens when a plant dies. It leaks energy. The healers in her experiment stimulated the dying leaves to leak energy faster so they would glow brighter. Under the lens of the bio-photon imaging system – the same kind used by scientists to observe faint distant stars – the leaves treated by the healers glow noticeably brighter.

Wondering what the super-skeptics would say, skeptics who claim healers are just hypnotists, Connor said, "How do you hypnotize a leaf?"

Good point. Even super-skeptics might have trouble claiming a leaf could be hypnotized, or fooled into believing it feels better. They would, however, likely allege some other kind of fraud.

Connor also pointed out earlier experiments at the lab by healers who worked with e-coli bacteria. The experiments, repeated over and over, showed dramatic growth in the e-coli treated by healers as opposed to e-coli in the control sample under very tightly controlled lab environment. "What would the super-skeptics say about that?" she asked. "Surely no one could say the e-coli were influenced psychologically or hypnotized by the healer, would they?" Good question.

Connor said they also used the imaging system to look at the healer's hands when they are running energy. Guess what – they glowed, very faintly, but the images clearly brighten when healers "run energy" – another indication that could link healer's energy with oscillating capillary blood flow or muscle movement.

Returning to the plants for a moment, the plant used in her experiments grows in the back corner of Dr. Connor's small office. It's thriving, as it should be in the presence of so many healers. But that wasn't always the case. When they began running the experiments, many of the healers broke down crying. They said they couldn't continue to harm the plant, claiming the plant was upset by the way the experiments were being done.

Connor was startled. "We had a series of healers who broke down crying," she said. "Saying they couldn't do this anymore. They said the plant wants you to restructure the study, and this is the protocol it wants you to use." She said the plant actually wrote the protocol that they eventually settled on.

But that's not all. "The healers did not know each other," Connor said. "They were kept completely separate, no contact, and they gave us exactly the same information…absolutely stunning."

The plant told several different healers - who had never met - the exact same thing. Among other things, the plant wanted Connor to clip leaves from the bottom of its stem, the leaves that were older. "The plant said you can use healthy or non-healthy leaves, but you need to cut the leaves that are older and more stable. It was a more natural process to what plants did, and as you can see," she said as she pointed toward her very healthy plant, "the plant is doing quite well."

The same information from so many different healers "kind of freaked me out," Connor said. "From that point forward, the experiments completely failed until we changed the protocol, then it worked just fine."

But the experiments may have created more questions than answers. Connor said, "So now, do we have non-human communication going on at a level we don't understand?" The lab also measured and photographed strings of energy flowing from one plant leaf to another. Are the plants communicating by "running energy?" Just another issue the lab hopes to investigate further someday.

Like nearly every scientific endeavor, the work at the lab will only go as far as its funding will take it. And few conventional sources of funding for scientific research will even look at this kind of work. Most of the healers taking part in her studies volunteer their time for a week or more; an expensive proposition for people who are generally self-employed.

In no way does Connor or anyone else at the lab believe energy healing can replace traditional medicine. But by combining the best both have to offer, it could make a difference in a lot of people's lives.

"Energy medicine might be able to strengthen existing western medicine," Connor said. "You don't throw out the baby with the bathwater. What western medicine does well, it does superbly. I'm kind of an 'everything the road will bear' kind of person," she added, "because people are works of art. One person may need help in the form of acupuncture. Another may need chiropractic. One person may need it in the form of meds, while another may need it in the form of surgery. There are many different paths to get to the same place."

Connor, who was born in New England, is a born clairvoyant. It took her years to realize she was different from other people. Healing wasn't her first passion – as a young woman she wanted to star on stage. Song and dance is her true passion, and she has an undergraduate degree in English and Directing.

Later in life, a hormonal imbalance caused something called Luteal Phase Deficiency – she kept losing babies in the first trimester of pregnancy. But after lots and lots of careful work, she was given a daughter, "now fifteen going on seventy," Connor joked.

Looking for ways to get pregnant and stop the migraine headaches that had tortured her since the age of twelve, led Connor to investigate alternative healing methods. She started training for massage therapy, because it provided relief for her migraines. And while taking part in Buddhist chanting, she could see her energy fields change – manipulating her own energy fields became a way to stop the hemorrhaging which had ended so many pregnancies.

But it was while she performed massage therapy on others that she began to notice improvements in her clients that couldn't just be attributed to massage. They were healing. "I didn't know that I could do the energy work initially," she said. "I didn't know that I'd been doing it basically without knowing it for years."

Connor added, "When I started doing massage work I realized my hands got hot, and I started to explore what that meant."

Wanting to know more about controlling her own pain led her to more energy healing study. Her family history helped her as well. "My mother was a physician," Connor said. "She taught residents. My father was a psychologist who worked at

348

Harvard and a number of other places. So we had medical types running through the house on a regular basis. I was constantly exposed to medical issues."

Connor began her practice as an energy healer in 1987, and has been doing it ever since. "It was surprising the level of comfort I had when I started to go into hospital settings. They were just like home. My first hospital experience was actually at eight weeks. My mom took me along when she went in to do therapy on people."

Being in so much pain herself, Connor felt the need to do something. "People by and large are in so much pain. It's not fun for them, and it's not fun to be around them."

The science of medicine only produced frustration for her. She knew that there had to be something more. There had to be another option. "I just watched the science throughout the years," she said, "and got more and more frustrated. Here, I was having results on my table. I'm watching bones fuse so that when the person goes back and brings in the next set of x-rays to his doctor, he can't see where the break was. And science was saying it wasn't real. I was watching my own body do it, and other people do it, so what's going on here?"

As for her work at the University of Arizona lab, Dr. Connor says, "We are missioned to find mechanisms of action in the healing process, specifically in energy healing but in healing in general as well." She says their mission is to promote the health and healing of the Earth and its people. "And when I say people, I mean all people."

She says, "I want to find out what the truth is. If I am crazy, I need to know that. If I am living in a fantasyland when I saw people get off the table who had come in a wheelchair, then I need to know that. If it's just placebo effect, then how can we stimulate the placebo effect?" She admits that placebo effect is an obvious factor when working on people, "but it's not a factor when I'm working on a leaf," she said. "There is something more that's going on, and we need to know what that something is.

"We are living in an unhealthy world," she said. "We are destroying our world extremely rapidly, and we don't get it. We are so stuck on survival mode. Did the kids get picked up time, did the clothes get cleaned? The mechanics of daily living are such that we can't get past that. We get bogged down by it. We may get moments where we can come up for air, but most people are bogged down. So the question is, how do we shift things? How do we create an environment that focuses on healthy living and healthy processes?"

But will energy healing ever be accepted by mainstream medicine? Connor thinks so, given time. "Chiropractic is becoming more and more mainstream," she said. "Acupuncture is becoming more and more mainstream. Seven point four billion dollars was spent out of pocket by American consumers on energy healing in 2004."

Still, Connor says she's not sure what the lab will be able to prove to everyone, especially the skeptics. She said, "In terms of what we'll prove, I don't know what we are going to prove."

But the data keeps growing. Part of her work includes studying electro-magnetic fields with a simple hand held electrical device originally designed for measuring electro-pollution. It's called a 3-axis digital Gaussmeter. It is normally used by electricians to find electric wires hidden behind walls or in ceilings. It measures extra low magnetic fields generated by electrical current.

Playing around with it one time, Connor discovered that when she "ran energy" the device registered a change in the magnetic fields around her hands. She then tried it out on the healers she was using in her study. Connor and her colleagues found that when they tested other healers, they found "highly significant increases in extra low frequency activity, replicated in both hands, over two trials."

Just another piece of the puzzle.

"We're just starting to explore," Connor said, "and we're talking about very minute changes in the energy field structure. Why minute changes would have as big an impact as they do physiologically we don't yet understand. That is one of the things that has yet to be addressed."

Stay tuned.

Chapter Sixteen
The Prophecies

On September, 11th, 2001, Jerry Wills turned forty-eight-years old. As America was under attack, Jerry realized it was a prophecy unfolding…a prophecy he was given years before.

Remember when you read about "M" and other entities that seemed to guide Jerry through his life? More than ten years before September 11, 2001, Jerry Wills had been told by these same entities to expect major changes, and that he needed to pay careful attention to world events. It was in early 1991, before his thirty-eighth birthday, that Jerry was warned about the period of time starting in 1991--that during this period there would be great changes. He had been warned about great Earth changes as early as his teenage years, but they were never as specific. "They said that, 'When the world goes to Riyadh, that the time had come for great changes,'" Jerry said. He also said that at the time, he knew nothing about Riyadh (The capital of Saudi Arabia). He said he didn't even know what the word Riyadh meant.

But it would soon come to his attention. In early 1991, the United States led a coalition of countries gathering forces in the Saudi Arabian desert near Riyadh to challenge Saddam Hussein's-led Iraqi takeover of Kuwait. "When Desert Shield started," Jerry said, "there was this newspaper headline that said 'The World goes to Riyadh.' And it just freaked me out. There really was a place called Riyadh. I'm looking at this and going, oh my God. I'm trying to live a normal life at this point. I'm not doing healings, not doing anything really, just work, work, work and trying to have some fun. But now, it was right there: The World goes to Riyadh. And from that point forward, I'm paying close attention to world events."

The last time Jerry heard from one collective he was in contact with was about ten years before 9/11/01. He hasn't heard from this specific group since, which is something disquieting for Jerry. "I guess that chapter is closed," he said. But the earlier prophecies stay with him. "They said that when the World goes to Riyadh is when the great changes have started and it will continue to escalate until the end of the cycle."

Many modern-day historians and analysts have linked what happened in 1991 and our current troubles with Islamic extremists. The late Osama bin Laden announced his Fatwa against the West, and in particular the United States, only after the Saudis refused bin Laden's offer to help fight off Iraq in 1991, and invited the United States and its allies to protect the Kingdom instead. It was only after the 1991 war that bin Laden and his loose confederation of Fedaheen fighters merged into "Al Qaeda," or, "The Base" that we are all so familiar with today. Before that, bin Laden had been best known for his fight against the Soviets in

Afghanistan, a fight supported by Washington and the CIA. But now with so many "infidels" occupying the holiest land of the Muslims, the protectors of Mecca and Medina, bin Laden turned his vengeful version of Islamic extremism on the West. The result has been attacks on U.S. Embassies in Africa, the near sinking of a U.S. warship and the attacks on 9/11/01, to name just a few. It has also led to the U.S. and U.N. occupations of Afghanistan, where al Qaeda and the Taliban remain a threat, and to a prolonged war in Iraq, where al Qaeda continues to flourish after the U.S. withdrawal.

Add to all that, the winds of war blowing toward a potentially nuclear armed Iran, and the chaos left over by the so called "Arab Spring," it adds up to a world looking more and more to be in a disastrous transitional state with no end in sight.

Just take a look at the technological war machine the United States has unleashed on most of the Middle East. Guided-missile armed drones seek out al Qaeda targets hiding in caves in Afghanistan and the tribal areas of Pakistan, killing hundreds. But have these computerized marvels brought us any closer to a peaceful conclusion?

On a larger but more common scale, take a look at people in the grocery store, or at those people driving their cars to work every morning. Chances are, at least half of them will be on their new smart phones or tablets. When they get home at night, stressed out over a long day in front of their workplace desktop computers, or from a commuter flight with their laptop battery drained, the first thing they do is turn on their fifty-four inch flat screen plasma TVs, or play mind-numbing video games full of violent action or war-game scenarios.

As I write this book's final chapter, a brand new chapter in the life of Jerry and Kathy Wills is just beginning. They now travel widely across the U.S. to hold healer sessions and take part in lecture tours. But they've also established a home base in Jerome, Arizona. Once a thriving copper mine boom town, Jerome is now a colony of artists and hippies, like Jerry. He and Kathy love the vibe there. Whatever the future holds, Jerry believes in God's plan for us all, something that's not easy for everyone to see. But alongside the dire predictions for the near future, Jerry still wants to give people hope.

"Sometimes you get so frustrated, you're not even sure if God exists," Jerry said. "You wonder about it. You lose faith, you lose hope and you can't see the light. A mountain of anxiety or anger smothers you. You are completely in a perspective where you can't tell which way is up. Some people get into such a troubled perspective that they don't know which way to turn, so therefore they don't turn in any direction. They just stop. You know, they say if God was real, why doesn't he do something about this?

"Why it works the way it works, who knows? But maybe in God's plan it's been determined that I'm going to be the one who is standing there like a real live person, saying you know what, God is real and here's proof of it. And when that happens, it gives people a sense that God is still alive and still powerful and effective in their lives, maybe in ways they are not familiar with or in ways they never expected. But, the presence of God was always there; they just got a new perspective of what the presence is all about."

But why are Jerry and others like him the ones to heal us, to reassure us of something more to come than the technological world we live in?

"There are many of us who choose to come into life during this age," Jerry said. "We've been through this before and intuitively know the path quite well. It's during these times when people need to be reminded of their true nature and their connection to God. You never realize how much you need this connection until troubling times occur. We help by gently guiding the age forward through our presence and actions."

When it comes to living a pure and perfect life, Jerry claims we don't have to worry about it. "I think the whole realm of being in this powerful attribute, thinking of them as being pure as driven snow and without fault, is a bunch of malarkey. I think that anything that is alive has free will, and anything that is conscious and self-aware has free will. And sure, wisdom can guide your feet, can help you to choose a direction, but it doesn't mean it will always help you choose the right direction. I think anything that is self-aware has the opportunity for making a mistake, including angels and spirits."

It's up to you, the reader, to believe any of this; to believe anything Jerry says; to believe what many of his clients have claimed; to believe some of the healings described in this book; or to believe the research on alternative treatments. It's up to you to believe it, to trust it, to at least hope it might be true.

We all have to have hope, or why bother? Many people believe that Jerry is one of those people who provide others with hope. He takes away the pain, and fear, that come with sickness or injury. But only for those who want to take a chance on something different, something that is difficult to license and board certify after years of clinical testing.

Jerry Wills is a healer. And after what many people have witnessed and discussed with others, they believe he is the real thing. Even when it doesn't work, his sometimes reluctant contribution as an intuitive can heal the soul. Even when others call into question the healing work done by Jerry and others like him, he still provides many people with hope for the future, which is anything but certain.

Some believe alternative methods for healing, for communicating with life after death consciousness, for exploring other realms of existence will be part of our future on this Earth. With an open mind, anything is possible.

Whether it is scientifically measurable or just a series of fascinating anecdotal stories, a growing number of people worldwide have begun to think there is something to all of this. Maybe something wonderful.

For More information about Jerry Wills, and how to book an appointment: www.jerrywills.com

For more information about the author: www.rodhaberer.com

Printed in Great Britain
by Amazon

48027529R00215